# Easy-to-Swallow, Easy-to-Chew Cookbook

*Over 150 Tasty and Nutritious Recipes for People
Who Have Difficulty Swallowing*

Donna L. Weihofen, R.D., M.S.
JoAnne Robbins, Ph.D., CCC-SLP
Paula A. Sullivan, M.S., CCC-SLP

JOHN WILEY & SONS, INC.

Published by John Wiley & Sons, Inc., New York
Published simultaneously in Canada

Illustrations courtesy © 2002 Kathryn M. Kleckner
Design and production by Navta Associates, Inc.

This publication is designed to provide accurate and authoritative information in regard to the subject matter covered. It is sold with the understanding that the publisher is not engaged in rendering professional services. If professional advice or other expert assistance is required, the services of a competent professional person should be sought.

Wiley also publishes its books in a variety of electronic formats. Some content that appears in print may not be available in electronic books. For more information about Wiley products, visit our web site at www.wiley.com.

ISBN 0-471-20074-3

Printed in the United States of America

10 9 8 7 6 5 4 3 2 1

# Contents

# Preface

E njoyment of food and drink is essential to our quality of life. Be it fine food or comfort food, the choices we make with regard to eating are integral to defining ourselves, our needs, and our relationships. The pleasurable dining experience is a major source of satisfaction that is taken for granted by most of us.

In fact, as leisure time is increasing in the United States, and with the anticipated extended retirements of America's aging baby boomers, we can look forward to more opportunities to share mealtimes and participate in social activities that include eating, drinking, and being merry. However, one ability that we take very much for granted but that may be impaired as we age is the act of swallowing. Although swallowing is not often an activity we consciously think about performing, we swallow hundreds of times each day, day in and day out.

While we have known for some time that certain diseases and conditions, such as stroke or cancer of the mouth or throat may affect our ability to swallow, the recognition that the process of healthy aging can impact our swallowing is relatively new. Since the advent of Social Security, the average lifespan in the United States has increased by approximately twenty years. Those who live into their eighties and nineties often experience age-related changes in sensitivity to taste, temperature, and texture; find it takes a greater effort to swallow food or liquids; and face an increased risk of choking.

This book was conceived through interactions with thousands of patients and their spouses or caregivers—the many people we met every day for fifteen years who were being challenged with swallowing difficulty, yet maintained the desire to continue enjoying food. It also was a response to the hundreds of very healthy older people who served as subjects for our many research protocols and taught us that even if you are relatively physically fit at sixty or older, you may be coping with subtle swallowing and eating issues, because aging affects all parts of us—even our mouth and throat muscles!

Many of the ideas in this book received the "stamp of approval" from patients who tried them and may have even shared with us ways to improve them. It is our hope that the tips and recipes we provide will restore or enhance *your* dining pleasure.

There is no doubt that relieving hunger is fundamental. We hope this book will help you do so with confidence, appeal, and gusto. Bon Appetit!

# Introduction
## *Why This Book?*

One of the great joys of life is savoring good food. We love to eat, and we enjoy providing food to our families and friends. We take pleasure in making food look good and taste great, and the pleasure is doubled when someone really savors the food. But not everyone experiences this joy of eating. For some, the eating experience actually is somewhat unpleasant. Eating can be a problem instead of a pleasure for people who have difficulty chewing or swallowing foods.

Difficulties with swallowing and chewing can be the natural result of aging, or can be caused by certain diseases and conditions that occur at any age. Swallowing and chewing problems commonly occur with stroke, Parkinson's disease, multiple sclerosis, head injuries, cerebral palsy, muscular dystrophy, Sjögren's disease, scleroderma, motor neuron disease (Lou Gehrig's), Alzheimer's disease, and cancer of the mouth or throat. Also, as medical and surgical methods improve and provide cures for some diseases, the treatments themselves may cause swallowing difficulties. For instance, throat cancer may be cured by surgically removing a part of the throat that is malignant, yet such a cure may, more often than not, compromise swallowing owing to reduced airway protection. Swallowing and chewing can also be compromised during or after radiation therapy or chemotherapy. And it has been estimated that some two thousand medications available today may improve certain conditions but have a major side effect, called xerostomia, which is dry mouth due to reduced saliva, that makes swallowing, particularly the swallowing of dry food, extremely difficult.

Many of the underlying causes of changes in swallowing, including the normal slowing of mouth and throat muscles that occurs as part of the healthy aging process, begin somewhat insidiously. They are hardly noticed until a specific type of favorite food seems to always be "sticking in our throat" or causes choking when it seems to be "going down the wrong pipe." When this starts to occur more and more often, people may feel puzzled, embarrassed, even ashamed. What can be done to make the enjoyment of food easier?

We are three professional experts: a nutritionist, a clinician-scientist, and a swallowing clinician who have spent our careers helping people with swallowing difficulties. We have combined our areas of expertise so that this book not only addresses problems that may be associated with swallowing and their causes, but also offers numerous tips, hints, and strategies to improve the swallowing function. The bulk of the book provides more than 150 fabulous recipes that you and your friends will enjoy, whether or not swallowing is a challenge.

So that you know a little more about us and our backgrounds, Donna Weihofen is a senior nutritionist at the University of Wisconsin (UW) Hospital and Clinics. Ms. Weihofen, R.D., M.S., lectures throughout the country and has written three popular books: *The Cancer Survival Book*, *Magic Spices*, and *Mom's Updated Recipe Box*. She is considered an expert in the field of nutrition.

Dr. JoAnne Robbins is an associate professor in the Department of Medicine and serves as associate director of the University of Wisconsin Institute on Aging and associate director of research of the Geriatric Research Education and Clinical Center at the William S. Middleton Memorial Veterans Hospital. She also directs the University of Wisconsin/Veterans Administration Swallowing Research Laboratory. Dr. Robbins has received federal research support from the National Institutes of Health and the Department of Veterans

Affairs for her entire career, which has been dedicated to swallowing and its disorders. Her work focuses on increasing the understanding of swallowing processes in patients who suffer from stroke, dementia, or Parkinson's disease in particular, and frailty more generally, as well as the effects of the healthy aging process on the swallowing mechanism and its function. She has authored over sixty publications in peer-reviewed journals and books.

Paula A. Sullivan, M.S., CCC-SLP, has specialized in swallowing rehabilitation for the past twenty years. Ms. Sullivan is a speech pathologist at the William S. Middleton Memorial Veterans Hospital in Madison, Wisconsin. She also has a faculty appointment as a clinical instructor in the Department of Surgery, Division of Otolaryngology, University of Wisconsin-Madison Medical School. Her publications include a textbook on swallowing problems in cancer patients.

We conceived this book in response to the thousands of patients we have cared for through the Swallowing Programs at the University of Wisconsin and William. S. Middleton Memorial Veterans Hospital. It also has been designed in response to the hundreds of healthy, vibrant older men and women who have taught us about some of the subtle— and not-so-subtle—swallowing changes that accompany relatively healthy aging, even in the best of circumstances.

This book will help the many people with swallowing problems who want to know what they can eat and drink *that they will be able to enjoy*, despite their swallowing difficulties. For, when swallowing and chewing are impaired, one's choices and desire for food become limited.

This book also will help the many spouses, partners, family members, care providers, and health care workers who wish to nurture someone in one of the oldest and most basic of ways—by providing nourishment, not merely for sustenance, but in a form that appeals to the senses and enhances quality of life.

It is our hope that this book will stimulate the palates of those who are currently limited, bored, or frustrated by their (or their loved one's) swallowing and chewing challenges. But bear in mind that while our intent is to enhance the dining experience by providing strategies and recipes for easy, safe, and enjoyable nourishment, this book is not a replacement for consultation with medical providers when dysphagia (difficulty swallowing) is suspected. Swallowing interventions should be provided by various health care professionals. When seeking the assistance of such an individual, it's important to verify the experience and training he or she has in the specialty of swallowing and swallowing disorders.

❖

# PART ONE

# Understanding Swallowing and Swallowing Difficulties

# How We Swallow

Most of us never think about swallowing until we get a bit of food or a pill caught in our throat, or until a sip of liquid "goes down the wrong pipe." However, swallowing is a highly complex balancing act. Approximately thirty mouth and throat muscles and multiple nerves must perform their actions precisely on cue. To understand this properly, let us look more closely at the aerodigestive tract, which comprises the mouth, throat, larynx (airway entrance), and upper esophagus (see Figure 1).

The aerodigestive tract channels air for breathing. In breathing, the air must move from the nose or mouth into the larynx. It then goes into the lungs and back and out. If you choose to speak, the air moves the same way through the aerodigestive tract, but the vocal folds then must vibrate to produce sound.

In order for you to swallow, the aerodigestive tract becomes an effective food propelling mechanism. The tongue propels food into the throat, which sends the food on to the esophagus so that it can be digested. However, during its transfer from mouth to esophagus, the food temporarily sits right next to the larynx and trachea (windpipe), which lead directly to the lungs. The epiglottis is responsible for covering the airway entrance to protect it from the presence of the food, and the larnyx itself moves out of the path of the food. The vocal folds also close to protect the trachea and lungs from this foreign material (see Figure 2).

This is a precarious situation, however. Occasionally, a piece of solid food can inadvertently go down "the wrong pipe," that is, the windpipe. Unless very small in size, this food can then block the airway, causing an inability to breathe.

The same thing can happen with liquids or soft foods, too. Entry of food or liquid into the trachea is called aspiration. If this occurs

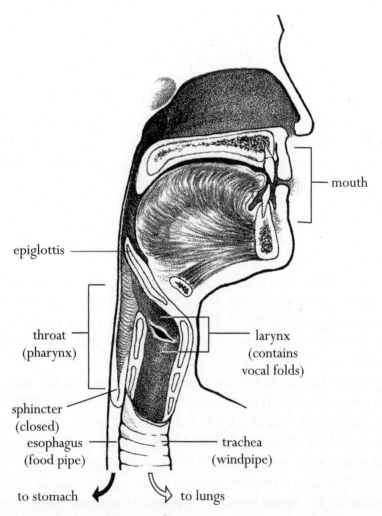

**Figure 1.**    The aerodigestive tract *(courtesy of Kathryn M. Kleckner)*

repeatedly, it can result in pneumonia or other types of damage to the lungs. When food, liquid, or saliva finds its way down the wrong pipe, it eventually will reach the lungs unless it is coughed out of the airway and expelled through the mouth.

The manner in which we normally swallow does not permit us to inhale food into our trachea and lungs. In fact, swallowing is one of the few acts we humans perform during which we must stop breathing. When we swallow, the larynx, which sits on the top of the airway

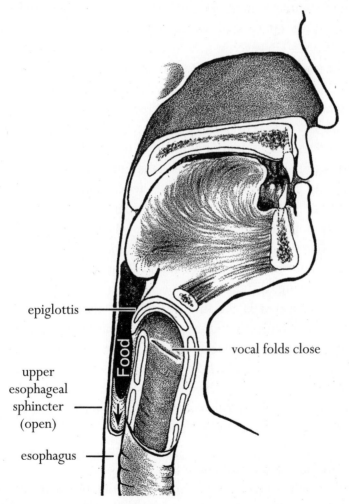

epiglottis

vocal folds close

upper
esophageal
sphincter
(open)

esophagus

Food

**Figure 2.**    Food moving through the aerodigestive tract *(courtesy of Kathryn M. Kleckner)*

on the trachea, is closed, and simultaneously the sphincter at the top of the esophagus (which is closed when we are not eating or drinking so that we do not swallow air) is opened for food passage toward the stomach (see Figure 2). These events, which must be timed precisely to the millisecond, are performed automatically by each of us approximately five hundred times per day.

Certain foods and liquids are easier or more difficult to swallow. Thin liquids, for instance, are most frequently aspirated because they can easily flow into a small opening, which is what occurs when the vocal folds at the top of the airway do not come together in a perfectly uniform manner. However, it is believed that thicker liquids are less likely to be aspirated. Although it is not clear why, the thought is that they offer increased *viscosity*. Viscosity is a property related to thickness and the manner in which a liquid flows. Viscosity is assumed to provide airway protection through increased sensory feedback, increased cohesiveness, and/or slowing of the liquid flow.

In terms of solid food, those foods that are dry and granular are most likely to cause aspiration. In fact, foods that do not maintain cohesion (that is, while in the throat, fall apart into little dry pieces, like rice or popcorn) may "particle-ize," thereby slipping easily through a narrow opening, or they may be inhaled easily.

In addition to the possibility of food or liquid being misdirected *during* swallowing, difficulty may occur because food stays in the mouth or in recesses in the throat that can "pocket" food. These recesses provide anatomic hiding places, so that after swallowing is completed, and breathing is resumed, the material is inhaled into the airway from those recesses where it has been stuck or pocketed.

It has become clear that certain consistencies of food and liquid appear to be easier or safer to swallow. These include soft, easy-to-chew items such as cooked vegetables or canned fruit; moist foods; and thicker liquids. These are the types of foods that you will soon discover are suggested throughout this book.

Now that we understand a bit more about the intricacies of swallowing and aspiration, let's look more closely at the ways in which you can make swallowing easier.

# 2

# Swallowing Safely and Easily

D ysphagia, or difficulty swallowing, has been estimated to affect approximately 15 million Americans. Approximately three thousand adults die every year because food gets stuck in their throats and blocks their airways, making it impossible to breathe. This occurrence is so common that it has been nicknamed the "café coronary." There is also the danger that food or liquid may enter the lungs, and result in recurrent infections or aspiration pneumonia. To reduce these risks, follow the guidelines and precautions listed below. These safe swallowing suggestions apply to everyone, with or without swallowing or chewing problems.

- Be aware of your posture. Eat sitting upright in a chair that provides adequate support. Avoid eating in places that have the potential to compromise your posture and safety, such as a recliner, bed, or car.

- Eat in a quiet, comfortable environment, free of distractions; for example, turn off the television.

- If you wear dentures, glasses, or hearing aids, or require any devices to support your head or neck, make sure to wear them when eating and drinking. Make sure your dentures are clean and fit properly and securely in your mouth.

- Do not talk while eating, as this has the potential to open your airway to food or liquid. Be a good listener if you have company.
- Do not rush while eating or drinking. Completely finish swallowing before taking the next bite or sip.
- Limit the amount of food or liquids eaten in one bite or one swallow.
- Eat in the presence of someone who knows the Heimlich maneuver, and know how to reach local emergency authorities quickly.

If swallowing or chewing is difficult, some additional specific principles should be observed. They are described in greater detail in the remainder of this chapter.

A word of caution: *no two individuals are alike in their swallowing or chewing problems*. A custom-tailored oral feeding program should be developed after a careful, detailed evaluation by an experienced team of health care professionals or a swallowing expert. Using the information from the swallowing evaluation, the experts can recommend strategies and plan a treatment determined to be the most appropriate.

# Posture and Position

Correct positioning of the head, neck, and body is critical to ensure safe swallowing, prevent choking or aspiration, and aid in digestion. The optimum posture for most individuals is to have the body seated in an upright position, with the head and neck tucked slightly forward, toward the chest. This posture protects the airway by positioning it under the tongue and prevents food from spilling into the airway.

Eating in bed should be avoided, but if it must be done, elevate the head of the bed in order to let gravity help the swallow. Or, position pillows to support the body and head in an upright position.

A person with a swallowing problem will require a posture or position specific to his or her swallowing needs. Postural techniques have been found to be effective in eliminating food entry into the airway in up to 80 percent of individuals with swallowing problems. Each posture must be carefully selected and evaluated by a swallowing therapist.

# Reflux Precautions

Prevention or control of gastroesophageal reflux (GER), which is the return of food upwards, is of special concern in individuals with swallowing problems. The esophagus is a long muscular tube that connects the mouth to the stomach. In the lower part of the esophagus, just above the stomach, there is a ringlike muscle that acts like a fist. The muscle is a one-way system that relaxes to allow food to pass on to the stomach, as well as to prevent stomach contents from moving upward into the esophagus, throat, or airway. Chronic reflux can cause problems such as chronic cough, hoarseness, difficulty swallowing, or damage to the vocal folds. Severe reflux can cause respiratory problems such as asthma, or, if stomach contents get into the airway, recurrent pneumonia. Common treatments include both lifestyle adjustments and medication. Over-the-counter medications may be helpful to treat the more common symptoms of reflux, such as heartburn. Other medications may need to be prescribed by a physician to neutralize or inhibit the production of stomach acid, or to improve emptying of the digestive tract. In severe cases of GER, surgery may even be necessary. However, most people with gastroesophageal reflux can be treated effectively with a combination of antacids and lifestyle modifications. These lifestyle modifications include changing posture, modifying diet, and changing eating habits. Common suggestions to control gastroesophageal reflux include the following:

- Be aware of your tolerance to tomato-based foods, highly spiced foods, fried foods, processed meats, citrus fruits, and fruit juices.

- Eat small meals high in protein and carbohydrates. Large meals are more likely to cause reflux problems.

- If possible, avoid eating, drinking, or taking pills less than three to four hours before going to bed or lying down.

- Limit intake of caffeinated coffee, colas, and fizzy beverages.

- Avoid or reduce intake of alcohol.

- Cut down or quit smoking.

- Lose weight, if needed.

- Avoid wearing tight-fitting clothing such as pants or pantyhose with tight waistbands.

- Don't exercise too soon after eating. Avoid activities that increase pressure on the stomach, such as bending over or lying on your side.

- Take medications two hours before lying down.

- Raise the upper body 6 to 8 inches by putting blocks under the head of the bed frame to raise it. Avoid placing additional pillows under your head as the subsequent bending of the waist and change in body position may increase abdominal pressure.

- Talk to your doctor about medications that may promote reflux or cause esophageal irritation or tissue injury. These include aspirin, ibuprofen, sedatives, tranquilizers, some antidepressants, and calcium channel blockers. Do not discontinue a needed medication without consulting with your physician.

## *Eating and Drinking Aids*

Eating and drinking aids can assist in placing, directing, or controlling the bolus (a cohesive mass) of food or liquid, and maintaining proper head posture while eating. For example, use of modified cups with cut-out rims (placed over the bridge of the nose) or straws will prevent a backward head tilt when drinking to the bottom of the cup.

A backward head tilt, which results in neck extension, should be avoided in most cases. When the head is tilted backward, food and liquids are more likely to enter the airway. Spoons with narrow, shallow bowls or glossectomy feeding spoons (a spoon developed for moving food to the back of the tongue) are useful to individuals who require assistance in placing food in certain locations in the mouth. More important, these utensils and devices promote independence in eating and drinking. A swallowing expert can make suggestions regarding appropriate aids for swallowing problems. Also, a partial list of companies offering these and other commercially available products can be found in Appendix B.

## *Oral Hygiene*

Proper oral care is essential, as the bacterial makeup of saliva can be changed through reduced or weakened swallows, dental disease, or malnutrition. Such altered saliva aspirated into the lungs, either before or after it is mixed with food or liquid, can increase the likelihood of infection or aspiration pneumonia. So perform the following oral care procedures on a daily basis:

- Oral care should be performed several times each day, ideally in the morning and prior to bedtime.
- A toothbrush or clean mouth sponge should be used to gently brush the teeth and tongue surface.
- Dentures should be cleaned, with a commercially available product after removal and prior to insertion. They also can be soaked daily in a 3 percent hydrogen peroxide solution.
- Excess saliva and food residue should be removed by a method recommended by a doctor, nurse, dentist, or swallowing expert.
- Dental examination and cleaning should be performed twice yearly.

- A whitish coating on the surface of the tongue is a sign of yeast growth. The doctor can prescribe a daily antifungal product to eliminate this problem.

- A partial list of commercially available products to relieve mouth dryness and soreness, as well as alcohol-free mouth care products can be found in Appendix B.

## Food and Liquid Rate and Amounts

In contrast to the "fast food society" in which we live, individuals with swallowing and chewing problems take longer to eat because of weakened muscles. Because of the increased length of time necessary, many people do not eat enough. The resulting fatigue then compromises swallowing safety. However, the optimum time needed to eat safely still is not known, because every individual and situation differs. Likewise, the amount of food or liquid needed to initiate a prompt and safe swallow varies. Typically, smaller amounts are less likely to enter or block the airway, but in individuals who experience a sensory loss to the mouth or throat after illness or injury, larger amounts of food or liquid may be necessary to trigger a swallow. To promote a safe and efficient swallow most individuals with swallowing and chewing difficulty should do the following:

- Always eat slowly and carefully. Allow adequate time for each meal. Do not eat or drink when feeling rushed or tired.

- Take only small amounts of food or liquid in your mouth. Use a teaspoon rather than a soup spoon. Take no more than one half to one teaspoon of food or liquid at any one time.

- Concentrate on swallowing. Hold the food or liquid in the mouth. Think about swallowing, and then swallow.

- Finish swallowing and relax before taking the next bite.
- If a straw is used, take one sip at a time, hold it in the mouth, and then swallow.
- Avoid mixing food and liquids in the same mouthful. Alternate solids and liquids. Avoid washing the food down.
- If there is weakness on one side of the face, place the food on the stronger side of the mouth. The head can also be tilted slightly to the stronger side to help the food pass into the throat.
- If lip muscles are weak and result in food falling out of the mouth, pinch the lips together with the fingers.

# *Medication*

Swallowing problems may affect an individual's ability to take medication safely and easily. In addition, the swallowing problem may interfere with medication absorption and effectiveness if the medication is consumed with inadequate amounts of food or liquid, or if taken incompletely. An individual who has difficulty swallowing thin liquids safely also will have difficulty swallowing thin liquid medications. On the other hand, pills or capsules may be particularly hard to swallow safely. Pill-induced damage to the esophagus can occur if pills are taken while lying down or with inadequate amounts of liquid. Certain pills can damage esophageal tissue if they are left in the esophogus to dissolve. Medicines also can enhance or interfere with the swallow. With certain disorders, such as Parkinson's disease, make sure that medication timing is monitored to allow the medicine to have its greatest effect at mealtimes. Many medications may cause dry mouth or esophageal dysmotility (inefficient esophageal function), which can interfere with the swallow. Consult with a doctor, pharmacist, or swallowing expert to help select medications that may be crushed, mixed with foods, or are available in liquid form.

# Mealtime Atmosphere

For individuals with a swallowing or chewing problem, eating and drinking no longer are easy, natural, enjoyable, or safe. Often, a sequence of strategies or compensations must be used in order to swallow more easily and safely. If the swallowing or chewing problem was caused by illness or injury, other problems, such as impaired memory or difficulty concentrating, also may be present. Therefore, a quiet, distraction-free atmosphere while eating is important to promote safe swallowing and enhance appetite and intake. Helpful strategies to allow the individual to concentrate on swallowing and chewing and enjoy mealtime include:

- Reduce noise and distractions, such as television, radio, pets, and telephone calls.
- In a restaurant, ask for a table away from the kitchen or doorway and in a corner.
- Limit conversation during the meal.
- Provide good lighting.
- Maintain small group dining.
- Keep the table setting simple by minimizing the number of items on the table. Remove salt and pepper shakers, and avoid table decorations.
- Be sure that foods are well-seasoned, flavored, and have an appetizing aroma to stimulate saliva production.
- Maintain a comfortable room temperature.

# Avoiding Choking, and Knowing the Heimlich Maneuver

Having a swallowing or chewing problem increases the risk of choking. Signs of choking include inability to cry out or speak, weak cough, grasping of the throat, labored breathing that produces a high-pitched noise, face turning blue, or loss of consciousness. The standard first aid technique to clear the airway is the Heimlich maneuver, or "hug of life." This maneuver involves standing behind the victim and wrapping the arms around the victim's waist. Next, a fist is pressed into the victim's stomach with a quick upward thrust and repeated until the object is expelled. Modifications are necessary if the victim is very obese, pregnant, a child, or an infant. Although the Heimlich maneuver can be self-administered, those with swallowing or chewing problems should always eat in the company of someone who knows this first aid maneuver. It is strongly recommended that family members be trained in emergency techniques for clearing the airway. Also, consider using an emergency service that can be called by the push of a button. Further information on the Heimlich maneuver can be obtained from the American Heart Association at (800-242-8721) or www.amhrt.org.

## *Recognizing Signs of Aspiration*

Certain warning signs may indicate the aspiration of food or liquid into the lungs. The changes listed below may occur, and if they do, they should be reported to the doctor and swallowing expert.

- Temperature spike or a low-grade fever for more than 24 hours. Temperature should be taken periodically and at approximately the same time daily.
- Increased coughing or choking.
- Changes in lung sounds.
- Increased secretions.
- More frequent upper respiratory infections or pneumonia.
- Weight loss.

Now let's examine the food textures offered in this book that should make swallowing easier.

# 3

# Tailored Food Textures and Nutrition Tips

Eating can be a pleasant part of life, or it can be frustrating. If eating becomes difficult because of chewing or swallowing problems, the delicious recipes and eating tips in this book can help bring the pleasures back. The recipes have been tailored to make food easier to chew and swallow, but they are such tasty recipes that they are sure to become favorites of the whole family.

The number one reason for choosing the recipes in this book is that the texture is tailored for you. Each recipe has a notation to let you know the characteristics of the recipe texture. Some recipes are for foods that are easy to chew with tender, small pieces of cooked foods. Some recipes are very easy to chew, with ground or mashed foods, and others are simply soft and smooth, with no chewing required.

Let's take a closer look at each type.

## *Easy-to-Chew with Mixed Textures*

### Description
- A wide range of texture mixtures may be served as tolerated. The textures can range from soft and smooth or mashed foods

to tender-crisp cooked vegetables. They can include ground meats and small pieces of tender cooked meat.

- All food should be tender.
- Food should be served in easy-to-eat pieces, although shapes and sizes of the pieces can vary.
- Food is soft enough so that it can be broken or mashed with a fork if needed.
- Meat and poultry is tender, moist, and well-done.
- Fish is free of bones, moist, and well-done.
- Fruits and vegetables are cooked or canned.

**To be avoided**

- Large pieces of food
- Nuts, seeds, popcorn, and chips
- Most raw or dried fruits and vegetables (unless they are very soft)
- Stringy or fibrous foods, such as pineapple, celery, leeks, pea pods, some green beans, and apple skin
- Tough or dry meats, poultry, or fish
- Whole grain breads with seeds or unground particles of grain
- Hard bread crusts
- Dry foods
- Foods with small dry particles
- Rice and other small grains (such as couscous) that are hard to control in the mouth
- Any food that is hard to form into a bolus (a cohesive mass of food or liquid)

# *Very Easy-to-Chew with Similar Textures*

## Description

- Foods are ground, minced, mashed, or cut up very finely.

- Foods should be moistened with gravies and sauces that will help in forming food into a bolus.

- Foods are soft enough to be managed well when teeth or dentures are not present.

- Vegetables are well cooked, chopped, or mashed.

- Fruits are soft, canned, or cooked.

- Meat, poultry, and fish are moist, well cooked, finely chopped, or ground.

- Small pieces of pasta are moistened with gravy or sauce.

- A bite of such food should contain only one texture. (For example, do not mix liquids with pieces of whole food, such as a broth soup with pieces of vegetables or meat.)

## To be avoided

- Mixed consistencies, such as minced foods in a watery broth

- Dry foods that could be inhaled, such as biscuits, crackers, chips, popcorn, hard bread crusts, or raw vegetables

- Whole grain breads

- Very sticky foods, such as peanut butter or sticky, gummy mashed potatoes

- Foods with skins or shells, such as peas, corn, or apple skins

- Tough, dry, or large pieces of meats, poultry, or fish

- Tough or firm foods that do not break down in the mouth or are difficult to manipulate
- Foods that are hard to form into a bolus, such as rice
- Large pieces of food
- Raw or crisp cooked vegetables and fruits
- Nuts and seeds
- Fresh salad greens

# *Soft and Smooth*

## Description

- Chewing is not required.
- All foods should be smooth, moist, and free of lumps.
- Texture can range from liquids to that of a jelly, mousse, flan, or pudding.
- Liquids may need to be thickened to a consistency to make them easier to swallow. The consistencies are described as: *thin*, *nectar*, or *honey* (the thickest consistency).

## To be avoided

- Foods that have crunchy pieces
- Foods that are fibrous or sticky, such as gummy mashed potatoes
- Foods with mixed textures
- Foods that are crumbly, such as scrambled eggs
- Foods and very thick liquids that stick around the mouth or are difficult to manipulate

- Foods that melt quickly in the mouth to a thin liquid, such as sherbets. (Thin liquids can trickle into the airway before you are able to swallow.)

- Dry foods such as breads, cereals, pancakes, or cakes that have been soaked in a liquid to soften

## Preparing Easy-to-Eat Foods

Preparing foods that are easy to chew and swallow may require some new cooking techniques and new kitchen equipment. The following information will make it easier for you to cook this way.

- If needed, any of the easy-to-chew foods in this book can be placed in a food processor and blended to the desired consistency. While any food can be chopped or puréed in a food processor, not all foods can be puréed in a blender. Blenders require a large amount of liquid to work properly.

- Food can also be blended in a cooking pan by using a hand-held immersion blender. This works especially well for soups.

- You also can process the foods just the way you like them. For example, you can leave the food lumpy and bumpy, which may be a bit more challenging to swallow, or make it soft and smooth, which is easier. Process foods to the consistency that works best for you.

- When blending hot foods, do not fill the blender or food processor more than one half full of hot foods or hot liquids. Place a towel over the top and pulse several times, very briefly, to prevent steam from causing the top to pop off.

- To thicken soups or stews, use potatoes, dried potato flakes, or mashed vegetables.

- Packaged gravy and sauce mixes are easy to use and make swallowing easier. Gravy adds flavor and moisture when puréeing meats. Sauces add flavor and moisture to vegetables and mixed dishes.

- Canned fruits are especially easy to purée. Place fruits in the food processor without the syrup and add the syrup gradually to make the desired consistency.

- Cooked or canned vegetables can be processed, too. Some vegetables need to be peeled before puréeing, including the stalks of broccoli and asparagus. If fiber remains in the puréed mixture, you may need to strain the mixture, then add enough liquid to make the desired consistency.

- If you are puréeing foods, try the following tip to make your plate more attractive. Keep a small amount of the whole food out of the food processor or blender. Place that whole food on the plate next to the chopped or puréed food. Having a garnish of whole food next to the puréed food may make your meal more appealing. However, if the whole food is too tempting, this will not be a useful strategy.

# *Meeting Nutritional Needs*

It is very important to make sure that nutritional needs are met if swallowing is difficult. Some people start limiting food variety and quantity because it is not easy to swallow, but enough protein and calories are essential for health and well-being.

## Protein

Protein is an important nutrient that is essential to every cell in the body: blood cells, brain cells, nerve cells, muscle cells, and so on. Sufficient protein must be included in the diet every day. To estimate your protein needs, take your weight and divide that number in half. That is a rough estimate of the recommended amount of protein for your body type. You do not have to count up the grams of protein that you eat each day, but if you are interested in estimating your intake, you can count up the grams in a typical day.

| | |
|---|---|
| 1 ounce meat, poultry, or fish | = 7 grams |
| 1 serving lentils, dry beans, or peas (½ cup) | = 6 grams |
| 1 cup milk (whole, 2%, 1%, or skim) | = 8 grams |
| 1 ounce cheese | = 6 grams |
| 1 serving bread products (1 slice) | = 2 grams |
| 1 serving pasta or rice (½ cup) | = 2 grams |
| 1 ounce tofu | = 2 grams |

If it is difficult to meet daily protein needs, try the following suggestions to increase the protein in your diet:

- Blend tofu into soups or main-course dishes. It is a great protein, and it will add smoothness to the dish without any unusual flavor.

- Mash or purée canned white beans (such as Great Northern beans) and add them to soups and main courses. They will add protein, fiber, vitamins, and minerals without any significant flavor.

- Add chicken broth to puréed white beans, and use it to moisten meat or chicken dishes.

- Add grated processed cheese to vegetable dishes.

- Add cottage cheese, ricotta cheese, or tofu to pasta dishes, casseroles, quiches, and egg dishes. For a smoother consistency, blend the cheese until smooth before using.

- Make creamy egg salad by finely chopping hard-cooked eggs, and adding mayonnaise, cream, mustard, garlic powder, salt, and pepper. Extra-firm tofu can also be added to the egg mixture. For a variation, add curry powder or finely chopped fresh herbs.

- Scramble eggs or liquid egg substitute with a bit of milk. Add grated cheese near the end of the cooking process to make a creamier, more cohesive egg dish.

- Add beaten eggs or liquid egg substitute to vegetable purées and sauces. Be sure to cook these dishes after adding the eggs.

- Add chopped or mashed hard-cooked eggs or tofu to casseroles, creamed meats, salads, and vegetable dishes.

- Choose dessert recipes that use eggs, such as bread pudding, rice pudding, custard, and other cooked puddings.

- Add instant breakfast powders to any milk-based beverage or food, such as cocoa drinks, milk shakes, and instant puddings.

- Use milk in recipes that call for water, such as instant cocoa, soup, bread or muffin mixes, hot cereal mixes, or pancake mixes.

- Add nonfat dry milk powder to foods such as cooked cereals, ground meats, casseroles, sauces, gravies, soups, dessert batters, and milk beverages.

- Add a commercial food enhancer to foods and beverages, such as casseroles, soups, sauces, muffins, cereals, mashed potatoes, coffee, and cocoa, without affecting the taste. One example is Nestle's Additions, which is a flavor-neutral food enhancer that adds 100 calories and 6 grams of protein per 19-gram scoop of powder.

# Calories

Calories are important, too. People with chewing and swallowing problems often have a hard time maintaining their weight. A person who is unintentionally losing weight is not eating enough calories. This can lead to significant muscle loss, increased risk of bone loss, and susceptibility to infections. When it is difficult to eat, it is important to choose foods that are packed with calories. These foods are often referred to as calorie-dense foods.

Most of the recipes in this book are fairly low in fat, although they are not so low in fat that taste is compromised. If extra calories are desired for weight maintenance or weight gain, you can easily substitute higher-fat ingredients. Just make the following substitution in the recipes:

| *Lower-calorie ingredient* | *Higher-calorie ingredient* |
|---|---|
| Fat-free milk | Whole milk |
| Fat-free or low-fat sour cream | Regular sour cream |
| Fat-free or low-fat cream cheese | Regular cream cheese |
| Low-fat cheeses | Regular cheeses |
| Low-fat mayonnaise | Regular mayonnaise |

# Other Ways to Increase Calories

### Eggs

- Eggs have 75 calories each and 1 cup of chopped, hard-cooked egg has about 100 calories.
- Add chopped, hard-cooked eggs to salads, vegetables, casseroles, and creamed meat dishes.
- Beat eggs or liquid egg substitute into mashed potatoes, sweet potatoes, vegetable purées, and sauces. Be sure to cook these dishes after adding the eggs; it is not safe to eat raw or under-cooked eggs.
- Add extra eggs to quiches, custards, puddings, pancakes, or French toast.

### Honey, jelly, and sugar

- These sweeteners have 50 to 100 calories per tablespoon.
- Add to cereals, milk drinks, yogurt, ice cream, and desserts.

- Use as a glaze for chicken or ham.
- Use extra amounts to sweeten foods and drinks.

## Salad dressings and mayonnaise

- Regular mayonnaise has 100 calories per tablespoon. Salad dressings vary in the amount of calories depending on the ingredients.
- Choose regular dressings and mayonnaise instead of reduced-fat dressings.
- Spread on sandwiches and crackers.
- Combine with meat, fish, egg, pasta, rice, fruit, or vegetable salads.
- Use in dipping sauces and gelatin dishes.

## Sour cream

- Regular sour cream has 30 calories per tablespoon.
- Add to cream soups, potatoes, noodle dishes, vegetables, sauces, salad dressings, and stews.
- Use as a sauce on cooked meats and fish.
- Use as a topping for cakes, fruits, gelatin desserts, breads, and muffins.
- Add some seasonings and/or herbs, and use as a dip for vegetables.
- Add a bit of brown sugar and mix with fruits.

## Light cream

- Light cream has 20 to 40 calories per tablespoon.
- Use in cream soups, sauces, egg dishes, batters, puddings, and custards.

- Pour on hot or cold cereals.
- Pour over fruits.
- Mix with pasta, rice, and mashed potatoes.
- Pour on chicken and fish while baking.
- Use as a binder in ground meats.
- Use to replace part of the milk in recipes.
- Use to make hot chocolate.

## Fats

- Fats and oils have 100 to 125 calories per tablespoon. Best for a healthy diet is olive oil or canola oil. Avoid margarines with trans fats, and limit other saturated fats in your diet.
- Add extra amounts to potatoes and other cooked vegetables.
- Use olive oil or melt butter or margarine as a dip for seafood, fish, meats, and vegetables.
- Add to soups.
- Add to gravies.
- Add extra amounts to eggs, pasta, rice, hot cereals, and grits.
- Combine with herbs and seasonings and spread on cooked meats, hamburgers, fish, and egg dishes.

## Ice cream

- Ice cream varies from 100 to 300 calories per ½-cup serving, depending on the brand.
- Use in beverages such as milk shakes and floats.
- Eat as a snack.
- Use as a topping for cereals, fruits, and desserts.
- Make ice cream sandwiches with graham crackers.

## Glucose polymers

- Commercial glucose polymers can be added to foods to increase calories without adding extra sweetness. They do not add any flavor or texture to the food. They contain fewer calories than the same amount of fat, but they may be helpful to use when you do not want the richness of fat. Polycose and Sumacal are two examples of commercial glucose polymers. They are in powder form and have 23 calories per tablespoon.
- Add the powder to cooked vegetables, casseroles, stews, desserts, and beverages.

## Commercial supplements

- Drink high-calorie nutritional supplements, such as Boost or Ensure, as needed, to help maintain or improve nutritional status.
- Carnation Instant Breakfast may be used as a supplement between meals. The most calories are gained by mixing it with whole milk. However, mixing it with 2%, 1% or fat free milk can also provide calories and nutrition.
- For a listing of available products see Appendix B.

These tips should make it easier to prepare foods that are nutritious *and* easy-to-swallow. The next chapter contains tips to help make swallowing easier.

# 4

# Tips for
# Easy Swallowing

Each person who is challenged by swallowing and chewing problems is unique. It is important to note that the tips offered in this
section will not apply to everyone. Use the tips if they can be helpful to make eating safe and more enjoyable for *you*.

## *"My Mouth Is Extremely Dry"*

Dry mouth, also known as xerostomia, is a side effect of many medications and chemotherapies. It can also be caused by radiation therapy to the mouth, head, or neck. When the salivary glands are altered
or destroyed, very little saliva is produced, or the saliva may become
very thick, sticky, and stringy. Saliva is one of those things you do
not appreciate until it is gone. Saliva moistens the mouth, and that
moisture helps you talk, eat, and swallow. It is critical to safe chewing and swallowing because it is difficult to form a bolus with your
food without saliva. Plus, it is difficult to keep food moving down the
throat and esophagus without the moisture and lubrication that saliva
provides. Saliva is also important for the health of the mouth. With
less saliva you are more prone to dental cavities and infections in the

mouth. A dry mouth may be a temporary problem, but in some cases it is a permanent condition.

**What to do**

- Ask your doctor to recommend a mouth-coating spray, wetting agent, or mouth cleanser. Some over-the-counter mouth moisturizers you may want to try include: Akolol Mucus Solvent and Cleanser, Biotene Dry Mouth Gum, Biotene Mouth Wash Antibacterial (alcohol-free), Glandosane Mouth Moisturizer, Mouth Kote Oral Moisturizer, Oral Balance Mouth Moisturizer, Stoppers 4 Dry Mouth Spray, Tung Gel Cleanser.
- Carry a squirt bottle or water bottle with you everywhere you go. Lemon juice mixed with the water may make it more appealing.
- Make your own mouth lubricant with a mixture of $\frac{1}{4}$ teaspoon of glycerin added to 1 cup of water.
- Chew sugarless gum or suck on sugar-free candy to stimulate saliva. Citrus-flavored candies, such as lemon drops, work best.
- Keep water by your bed for nighttime dryness.
- Rinse your mouth with a baking soda solution before and after meals. Mix $\frac{1}{4}$ teaspoon of baking soda in 1 cup of water. Do not drink the solution.
- Make stews, casseroles, and tender cooked foods with extra liquids to make them softer.
- Moisten foods with sauces, gravies, and dressings. Soften or thin foods with milk, broth, water, or melted margarine.
- Dip or soak foods into whatever you are drinking.
- Chop, grind, or purée foods. A small portable food grinder may be helpful.
- Drink liquids between bites of food.
- Choose fruits and juices that are low in acid, such as bananas, cooked apples, or canned fruits. Fruit nectars and fruit drinks

may be better tolerated than fruit juices. If nectars are too thick or too sweet, use club soda to thin them.

- Cool foods can be soothing. Suck on frozen juice bars, ice chips, or other cold foods if you are able to swallow thin liquids safely. Keep small pieces of fruit, such as banana pieces, melon balls, peach slices, fruit cocktail, and mandarin oranges, in the freezer, and suck or chew on the frozen fruit between meals.

- Choose smooth, soft, creamy foods like soup, macaroni and cheese, casseroles, canned fruits, tender cooked vegetables, puddings, custards, yogurts, or ice creams.

## Things to avoid

- Hard, crunchy foods or dry snack foods.
- Tough or crisp meats.
- Foods that gum up in your mouth, such as bread products and potatoes (unless very moistened) and other starchy items.
- Peanut butter on crackers, toast, or bread. If you absolutely love peanut butter, mix it with lots of honey, jam, or jelly.
- Spicy, salty, or acidic foods that can irritate your mouth.
- Hot food and beverages. Room-temperature foods are recommended.
- Caffeinated drinks. Caffeine may cause added dryness.
- Alcohol and tobacco. Tobacco can irritate the lining of your mouth and alcohol can make dry mouth worse.
- Commercial mouthwashes that contain alcohol. They can be drying and irritating to your mouth. Look for alcohol-free mouth-care products.

## Keep dental care in mind

- Visit your dentist often. With a dry mouth, you are at greater risk of infections, tooth decay, and more rapid plaque build-up.

- Clean your mouth and teeth often using a method recommended by your dentist.

- Avoid frequent intake of high-sugar drinks and foods, which promote tooth decay.

- Rinse your mouth whenever you feel you need to remove debris, to stimulate your gums, to lubricate your mouth, or to put a fresh taste in your mouth.

## *"My Mouth Is So Sore"*

Inflammation or sores in the mouth can make eating very difficult. It is important to find foods that you can eat with minimal pain and discomfort. Healing will occur more rapidly if you are eating well and drinking ample fluids.

### What to do

- Make your foods softer and moister.
- Sauce your foods. Add sauces, such as margarines, butter, gravy, cheese sauce, or cream sauce, to your meats and vegetables.
- Choose cool, soft foods such as mashed bananas and other mashed fruits, canned fruit, cottage cheese, soft-cooked or scrambled eggs, macaroni and cheese, custards, and puddings.
- Avoid alcohol, which irritates and dries the mucosa of the mouth and throat.
- Avoid spicy, hot, salty, or acidic foods such as pickles and vegetables marinated in vinegar.
- Increase fluid intake with water, nectars, cool soups, fruits, sherbets, and ice cream. Use a blender to make an icy slush with ice cubes and fruit.
- Eat in restaurants that feature buffet-style service where there is a variety of foods you can try in small quantities. You can add

sauces and liquids to the food at your discretion. It may be more comfortable for you to eat during the off-hours when there are not many other customers.

- Make a soothing, effective mouth rinse with one teaspoon of baking soda in one cup of warm water. Avoid mouthwash products that contain a large amount of salt, alcohol, or other irritating ingredients.

- Try holding a wet tea bag on the sore areas of your mouth to make it feel better.

- Use viscous lidocaine or oral analgesics before meals. These may be used only after their use is discussed first with your doctor or speech language-pathologist. They must be used with caution, as they can numb your swallow.

- Keep your mouth and gums clean to prevent infections. Check in with your dentist often. You also may want to try these over-the-counter products: Anbesol Oral Anesthetic, Kanka Mouth Sore Medication, Orabase Oral Anesthetic Paste, Oral B Amosan Oral Wound Cleanser, Orasol Anesthetic and Antiseptic, Proxigel CanKer Sore Relief, S.T. 37 Antiseptic Oral Pain Reliever, Ulcer Ease Antiseptic, Walgreen's Oral Analgesic Paste and Gel, Zilactin for Canker Sores and Cold Sores.

## "My Tongue Doesn't Work Too Well"

When there is limited range of motion or decreased sensation of the tongue, it is difficult to get food gathered together in the mouth to form a bolus. Forming food into a bolus is an important part of swallowing.

**What to do**

- Consult a swallowing expert who can recommend exercises to improve the range of motion of the tongue.

- When eating, tilt your head slightly to the side of your mouth or tongue that works better to use gravity to keep the food on that side for best manipulation.

- Tilt your head forward slightly (45° angle) so that food will not slip over the back of the tongue before your airway is protected.

- Experiment with different food consistencies. Soft, smooth foods eliminate the need to use the tongue to form a food bolus.

- Experiment with varying bite sizes to determine which sizes are easiest for you to swallow. Very small bites may be difficult to handle; large ones may result in an inability to keep it all in your mouth.

- Moisten food to help form it into a bolus.

- Drink a cold liquid between bites of food.

- To improve sensation, use a very cold spoon so you can tell where the food is in your mouth. To keep the spoon cold, place it in ice water between bites. The cold stimulation helps produce a swallow response.

- Press the spoon or utensil down firmly on the tongue when placing the food in order to increase sensation.

## *"I Have a Tongue Thrust"*

Tongue thrust is a movement of the tongue that pushes food out of and in front of the mouth instead of pushing food toward the back of the mouth. This interferes with the ability to eat.

### What to do

- Enlist the help of a swallowing expert to determine the underlying causes of your protruding tongue or the causes of involuntary tongue movements that expel food from the mouth.

- Eat very small amounts per bite, for example, ½ teaspoon per bite.

- Place food toward the middle to back of the tongue to facilitate bolus formation.
- Don't put in the next bite until the first bite has been swallowed.
- Put the food in through the side of the mouth rather than the front.
- If you need to swallow, gently touch your throat to initiate the swallow response.
- Do not rush. Allow plenty of time for swallowing.
- Alternate between liquids and solid foods.
- Choose moistened ground or smooth foods.
- Thicken liquids and thin purées to fit your need.
- Avoid dry foods, which are difficult to form into a bolus.
- Chew on the best side of your mouth if one side works better than the other.
- Try retraining exercises for the tongue. Push the tongue against the roof of the mouth or hold the tip of the tongue against the roof of the mouth just behind the top teeth and swallow with the lips open.
- Make sure you are sitting up straight, in good swallowing posture.

## *"Food Seems to Get Stuck in My Mouth"*

Some people have difficulty feeling when food is in their mouth or where it is in their mouth. If you have this problem, food may accumulate on the roof of your mouth or in the pockets in your cheeks.

### What to do

- Ask the pharmacist or doctor to review your medications. Some medications cause a very dry mouth and that may contribute to this problem.

- Add extra sauces and gravies to make food soft and moist.

- Alternate between liquids and bites of solid food.

- Soft and smooth foods may work best.

- Try to sweep the mouth with your tongue to clear food that stays behind. You can also use your finger to clear food from the roof of your mouth or from your cheek.

- Lean one side of your face (the side of your mouth in which food pockets) against your hand while you chew and swallow in order to keep the pocket closed to food.

- If one side of your mouth works better than the other, tilt your head to that side while chewing and swallowing so that gravity maintains the food or liquid on your better side.

## "I'm Always Trying to Clear My Throat, and I Cough When Eating"

Chronic throat-clearing, coughing, and choking are important signals that something is interfering with the swallowing mechanism. Persistent throat clearing is a subtle form of coughing and may be associated with silent aspiration. That occurs when small amounts of food get into the passages of the lungs and we don't feel or realize it. Other signs and symptoms of aspiration, whether silent (no cough) or not, are a wet voice quality or hoarseness. It is very important to find the cause of the problem before you continue to eat to prevent aspiration of food or liquid, since continued aspiration can lead to pneumonia or other types of damage to the lungs. A swallowing expert, usually a speech pathologist, will perform a swallowing X-ray (video fluoroscopic swallow study) to evaluate your swallowing mechanism and determine, along with your physician, the best treatment plan.

**What to do**

- Check with a swallowing expert to determine the best food consistency and liquid consistency for you.
- Be careful not to overfill your mouth when eating.
- Check your position when eating. Poor positioning can interfere with your ability to swallow. Remember, sitting upright (at a 90° angle) is usually the optimal position for eating.
- Ask for information on special eating techniques and eating utensils that may be helpful for you.

## *"I Feel Like I Have a Lot of Mucus in My Mouth and Throat"*

Excessive mucus or extra-thick mucus may be caused by respiratory infections, sinus infections, allergies, and dehydration. It is also a side effect of some neurological disorders such as Parkinson's disease or stroke, a side effect of cancer of the mouth or tongue, and a side effect of radiation to the mouth, head, or neck area. Also, it is often a sign that the swallow is weak or occurring less often than it should.

**What to do**

- Consult with your physician to resolve any infections that may be contributing to the abnormal secretions. Check on the possibility of allergies and use appropriate allergy medications if indicated.
- Try to clear secretions by providing humidification.
- Ask your physician or a swallowing expert about the possibility of suctioning to clear excess secretions from the airway.
- Avoid creamy and fatty foods that coat the mouth and throat.

- Choose skim milk instead of whole milk. It is important to know that milk does not cause mucus, but rather it coats the mucus you already have in your throat.
- Drink a small amount of cranberry juice or lemon juice mixed with water before eating or drinking to help clear the mucus.
- Choose clear, liquid, fruit-flavored supplements, such as, Enlive or Resource, instead of creamy supplements.

# *"Sometimes I Find It Difficult to Swallow Liquids"*

It is important to determine what form of liquid and soft foods you tolerate best. In this book, the consistencies of liquids are described as thin, nectar, or honey. Some liquids may need to be thickened to make swallowing easier, as more viscous liquids are often easier to swallow than thin liquids.

**What to do**
- Add thickeners to thin liquids to reduce the risk of the liquids getting into the airway. Some liquids and puréed foods can be thickened with unflavored gelatin, cornstarch, flour, instant mashed potato flakes, mashed vegetables, or cream of rice. There are also commercial thickening agents available. Some examples are: Thick-IT, Thick'n Ease, Thixx, Thickenup, Nutra-Thick, and SimplyThick.
- Commercially available thickened beverages include Resource Thickened Juice (of many flavors), Resource Thickened Water, Resource Thickened Coffee, and Resource Thickened Milk. They are all available in honey or nectar consistencies. Home delivery can be arranged through Novartis Nutrition (800-828-9194).

- Special cups have been designed to help swallow liquids. These cups allow you to drink without tilting your head back, helping you drink safely without aspirating the liquid (see Appendix B for suppliers).

- Avoid drinking with a straw. It is difficult to control the amount of liquid taken from straws, and straws tend to deposit liquid toward the back of the mouth, where it may easily enter the airway.

# *"I Get Full So Fast"*

Sometimes you may seem to fill up quickly, even though you used to be a big eater. It may take a lot of time and energy to eat, but it is important to maintain a healthy weight. You need to choose foods that are rich in nutrients and calories.

**What to do**

- Do not waste your time and energy eating foods that fill you up but don't have many calories or nutrients, such as broths or diet sodas.

- When choosing liquids to drink, select nutrient-dense fluids such as milk, milkshakes, juices, and punch-type drinks.

- Place only small servings of food on your plate so that eating a whole meal does not seem to be such an overwhelming or impossible task.

- Keep easy-to-eat snack foods readily available.

- Eat small amounts of food frequently.

- Limit the amount of fluids you drink with your meals. Liquids tend to make people feel full. Save the water, tea, coffee, and other liquids for between meals.

- For more ideas, see the section titled "Hints to Increase Calories" in chapter 3.
- If none of these suggestions work, you may be experiencing difficulty in your esophagus. When food is not pumped through the esophagus into the stomach efficiently or if food is returning through the esophagus from the stomach (reflux), a feeling of fullness is a common symptom. In this case, contact your doctor.

# *"I Get Tired Easily and Don't Have Much Energy"*

Fatigue may be experienced as tiredness, weakness, lack of energy, or sheer exhaustion. Learning to recognize and respect one's limits often means making adjustments in exercise, work, sleep, meal, and social schedules. Extra rest and nutritious food is important because inadequate intake of calories and other nutrients can compound fatigue. Adjusting eating schedules and food choices can help.

**What to do**

- Eat as much as possible at your best time of day. For example, if your fatigue worsens later in the day, eat a larger breakfast or lunch.
- You may feel more like eating after you have napped or rested.
- Eat many small meals and snacks throughout the day.
- Avoid skipping meals and snacks. Choose liquid nutritional supplements to replace a meal or snack if easy-to-prepare food is unavailable.
- At times when you have more energy, prepare foods in quantity. Refrigerate or freeze for later use.

- Keep meal leftovers in containers that can easily be warmed in the microwave.

- Use frozen or canned convenience foods that require little preparation.

- Purchase supermarket prepared foods and take-out food from restaurants.

- Accept offers of family and friends to help out. Let people know what foods work best for you.

- Consult with your doctor about adjusting medication schedules to optimize energy and function at mealtime.

- Check on availability of Meals on Wheels in your community.

- Check on the availability of a "take-out taxi" service in your area. This service will pick up food from participating restaurants and deliver it to your door.

# *"Food Just Doesn't Taste the Same"*

Medications, radiation, and some diseases can affect the taste buds in the mouth. Foods then can taste very different from what you expect, and sometimes they taste exceptionally bad. Some people experience a bitter or a metallic taste in their mouth. For others, food tastes "like nothing." And for some, taste preferences can change from day to day.

**What to do**

- Many foods, including meat or poultry, taste better if they are served cold or at room temperature instead of hot.

- Choose eggs (a good protein substitute) if you no longer like the taste of meat.

- Fresh fruits and vegetables, pasta dishes, and milk products are often well tolerated.

- Fruit sorbet, sherbet, and fruit smoothies usually taste good. Make your own frozen juice pops with your favorite juices.

- Tart sauces and condiments may be added to foods to help cover a metallic taste. Try adding orange juice, lemon juice, orange marmalade, pickles, seasoned vinegars, balsamic vinegar, and other seasonings to certain foods. If you do not have sores in your mouth, try using horseradish or any of the flavored mustards, as a condiment on your foods to add flavor.

- Rinse your mouth with fruit juice, wine, tea, ginger ale, club soda, or salted water before eating. This will help to clear your taste buds.

- You may sometimes be able to take away the strange taste in your mouth by eating foods that leave their own tastes in your mouth, such as fresh fruits or hard candies.

- Suck on lemon drops or mints, or chew gum after eating to get rid of undesirable tastes that linger.

- Try marinating meat or poultry in fruit juices, wines, vinegar-based salad dressings, or other sauces for more taste.

- Experiment with spices and herbs. Some people find they like spicier foods at this time.

- Experiment with new foods. Try foods or cuisines that you may not have tried before.

- Eat out in restaurants that feature buffets. You can try small amounts of a variety of foods to discover what foods taste the best to you.

- Check with your dentist to rule out any dental problems that may be causing a bad taste. Care for your mouth and teeth to prevent dental caries.

**Things to avoid**

- Do not force yourself to eat foods that taste bad. Instead, find substitutes for those foods. For example, if meat doesn't taste right, select chicken, turkey, fish, eggs, cottage cheese, cheese, eggs, yogurt, or tofu.

- Avoid eating canned soups or vegetables labeled "no salt added" or "low salt" (unless you have high blood pressure and are instructed to do so by your physician). Soups and vegetables tend to have a metallic taste when the salt has been eliminated.

- Do not drink citrus juices such as orange or grapefruit immediately after brushing your teeth with fluoride toothpaste. The chemical mixture of stannous fluoride with citric acid results in a rather unpleasant taste in your mouth.

- If a metallic taste in your mouth persists, avoid using metal dishes and utensils. Try using plastic eating utensils, chopsticks, or porcelain Chinese soup spoons.

- Avoid metal cooking utensils. Use wooden spoons, rubber spatulas, or plastic cooking utensils.

- Avoid cooking with shiny, thin aluminum cookware, copper cookware, or cast iron frying pans or pots. Metal flavor may transfer to the food, especially if the food is acidic. Choose stainless steel or Pyrex cookware instead.

- Stop smoking and drinking alcoholic beverages, which dull and distort your ability to taste foods. Alcohol also makes your mouth dry.

## *"I Have a Major Problem with Constipation"*

Problems with constipation are common when eating a soft or liquid diet. Constipation is also a common side effect of some medications, including pain medications. It may also result from inadequate fluid or fiber intake, or may be caused by a lack of exercise. To prevent constipation, drink lots of fluids and include more fiber in your diet.

Food and fiber work together. Fiber absorbs water in the intestine, to help soften and increase stool size, thereby promoting faster movement through the intestine.

## What to do

- Choose several servings of fruits and vegetables every day. You do not have to eat the fruits and vegetables raw to get the fiber. The fiber remains after cooking or canning or even if the foods are blended in the food processor.

- If you can eat bread, choose whole grain breads without seeds rather than more finely ground white breads or highly refined cereals. Examples include whole wheat, dark rye, pumpernickel, and oatmeal breads.

- High-fiber cereals include bran, shredded wheat, whole grain, bulgur wheat, and granola. Soak them in milk to soften them if it helps in swallowing.

- Add 1 to 2 tablespoons of 100 percent bran or wheat germ to your favorite cereal and to other foods.

- Try cooked dried fruits for snacks or desserts.

- Choose soups, salads, and main courses that use cooked dried or canned beans or lentils.

- Prepare dips and spreads from puréed canned beans, such as pinto, black, kidney, and garbanzo beans.

- Try prunes or prune juice for their laxative effect.

- If you are drinking a nutritional supplement, choose one with fiber added, such as Boost with fiber or Ensure with fiber.

- Commercial psyllium products are available and, if used regularly, can help to prevent constipation. This may be an essential and easy way to get enough fiber if you find that high-fiber foods are difficult to swallow.

- Commercial soluble fiber products, laxatives, stool softeners, and medications are also available. These include bulk-

forming products, such as psyllium-containing products—
Metamucil, FiberCon, and Citrucel; stimulants, such as Cor-
rectol, Ex-Lax, Dulcolax, and Senokot; stool softeners, such as
Colace, Dialose, and Surfak; and osmotics, such as milk of
magnesia, Lactulose, and Epsom salts. (Lubricants, such as
mineral oil, are not recommended because they cause significant loss of fat-soluble nutrients.)

### General Guidelines to Prevent Constipation

- Treat the underlying disorder.
- Develop good bowel habits.
- Drink plenty of fluids (8 to 10 full glasses each day).
- Try drinking a warm or hot beverage. This may help to stimu-
  late bowel movements.
- Exercise regularly. Take walks. Light exercise can stimulate
  bowel activity.
- Choose a well-balanced diet and enjoy relaxing meals.
- Gradually increase your intake of high-fiber foods. A reason-
  able goal is 25 to 35 grams of fiber per day. Check food labels
  for fiber content of specific foods, and note that the nutritional
  analyses of the recipes in this book provide the fiber content.
- Important: Check with your physician if constipation persists or
  if you notice thin, pencil-like stools, abdominal pain and bloat-
  ing, weight loss, or rectal bleeding.

# PART TWO

❖

# *The Recipes*

# APPETIZERS

❖

Black Bean Spread

Crab Horseradish Spread

Lemon Tuna Mousse

Liverwurst Pâté

Mushroom Spread

Oriental Shrimp Dip

Roasted Red Pepper and Bean Dip

Salmon Log

Salmon Mousse

*Note:* If it is difficult for you to eat breads and crackers with these dishes, try using a carrot stick or bread stick as a dipping utensil. Eat and enjoy the spread or pâté without the bread!

# Black Bean Spread

❖

*Choose any variety of canned beans, but be sure to use fresh cilantro. Make it as hot as you like it with cayenne pepper.*

❖ SERVES 8 ❖

Recipe texture: Soft and smooth

1   15-ounce can black beans,
    drained and rinsed
½   cup salsa, hot or mild
2   tablespoons lime juice
2   tablespoons chopped fresh
    cilantro

¼   teaspoon cumin
½   teaspoon sugar
salt to taste
cayenne pepper to taste
cilantro for garnish

Combine beans, salsa, lime juice, cilantro, cumin, and sugar in a food processor. Process until smooth. Adjust seasoning with salt and cayenne pepper to taste. Garnish with additional chopped cilantro. Spread on crackers or warm tortilla wedges.

NUTRITIONAL INFORMATION PER SERVING
Calories 55; Fat 1 gm.; Protein 3 gm.; Carbohydrate 9 gm.;
Cholesterol 0 mg.; Fiber 3 gm. (high)

# Crab Horseradish Spread

❖

*Serve this warm or cold with cocktail rye bread.*

❖ SERVES 8 ❖

Recipe texture: Very easy to chew

1  8-ounce package fat-free or
   low-fat cream cheese, room
   temperature
1½ teaspoons milk
½  teaspoon horseradish
dash white pepper

4  ounces canned or frozen crab or
   surimi seafood
salt to taste
dash garlic powder (optional)
dash Tabasco sauce (optional)

In a small bowl, combine cream cheese and milk. Mix until smooth.
Add horseradish and pepper. Mix well. Stir in crab. Add salt to taste.
Add garlic powder and Tabasco, if desired. Taste and add additional
horseradish, if desired. Place in small microwave-safe dish. Serve at
room temperature or warm briefly in the microwave.

NUTRITIONAL INFORMATION PER SERVING
Calories 35; Fat 0.2 gm.; Protein 6 gm.; Carbohydrate 2 gm.;
Cholesterol 30 mg.; Fiber 0 gm.

# *Lemon Tuna Mousse*

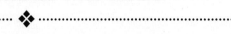

*Great as an appetizer or serve for a light lunch.*

❖ SERVES 6 ❖

Recipe texture: Soft and smooth

1   12-ounce can white tuna in
     water, drained
2   tablespoons butter or margarine,
     softened
1   teaspoon grated lemon rind
2   teaspoons lemon juice

⅓   cup extra virgin olive oil
1   teaspoon oregano
3   cloves garlic, chopped
dash Tabasco sauce (optional)
salt and freshly ground pepper to
     taste

Combine all ingredients except salt and pepper in food processor.
Process until smooth. Add salt and pepper to taste. Spoon into a
serving bowl. Refrigerate until ready to serve.

*Note:* Substitute other herbs of your choice for the oregano, if
desired.

NUTRITIONAL INFORMATION PER SERVING
Calories 220; Fat 17 gm.; Protein 15 gm.; Carbohydrate 1 gm.;
Cholesterol 35 mg.; Fiber 0.1 gm. (low)

# Liverwurst Pâté

❖

*If you like liver, you will enjoy this high-protein appetizer.*

❖ SERVES 10 ❖

Recipe texture: Soft and smooth

| | |
|---|---|
| 1  pound liverwurst | ¼  teaspoon onion powder |
| 4  ounces fat-free or low-fat cream cheese, room temperature | ¼  teaspoon garlic powder |
| | 1  teaspoon sugar |
| 1  tablespoon fat-free mayonnaise | 1  teaspoon chili powder |
| 1  tablespoon fat-free milk | |

**Topping**

| | |
|---|---|
| 4  ounces fat-free or low-fat cream cheese | dash Tabasco sauce |
| | dash garlic powder |
| 1  tablespoon fat-free mayonnaise | |

In a medium bowl, combine all ingredients except topping ingredients. Mix with a spoon until smooth. Spoon into pie pan and smooth the top with a flat knife.

In a small bowl, combine topping ingredients. Stir until smooth. Spread over pâté. Cover and refrigerate until ready to serve.

*Note:* The topping is optional. Instead of serving pâté in a pie pan, omit the topping and form the pâté into small, bite-size balls.

NUTRITIONAL INFORMATION PER SERVING

Calories 165; Fat 13 gm.; Protein 9 gm.; Carbohydrate 3 gm.;
Cholesterol 75 mg.; Fiber 0 gm.

# *Mushroom Spread*

......................... ❖ .........................

*Serve this superb blend of flavors to company
and be prepared to give out the recipe.*

❖ SERVES 10 ❖

Recipe texture: Very easy to chew;
Soft and smooth if blended

2   slices bacon, diced
1   pound fresh mushrooms, finely
    chopped
1   small onion, finely diced
⅛   teaspoon thyme
¼   cup sherry
1   8-ounce package low-fat cream
    cheese, at room temperature

1   tablespoon Worcestershire sauce
1   tablespoon soy sauce
½   cup fat-free sour cream
salt and freshly ground pepper to
    taste
dash Tabasco sauce to taste

In a medium skillet, cook bacon over medium heat. Add mushrooms,
onion, and thyme. Cook until mushrooms are tender. Pour off any
bacon fat that remains and discard. Add sherry and cook until liquid
is partially evaporated. Add cream cheese, Worcestershire sauce, and
soy sauce. Stir over low heat until blended well. Stir in sour cream
and heat through. Do not boil. Add salt, pepper, and Tabasco to taste.
Serve warm with crackers or toast pieces.

*Note:* For a smoother consistency, blend mixture in a food processor
until smooth.

......................

NUTRITIONAL INFORMATION PER SERVING

Calories 105; Fat 5 gm.; Protein 5 gm.; Carbohydrate 10 gm.;
Cholesterol 10 mg.; Fiber 2 gm. (medium)

# *Oriental Shrimp Dip*

❖

*This spread has a wonderfully subtle oriental flavor.
Serve it on crackers or chips for an appetizer,
or on toasted bread for lunch.*

❖ SERVES 12 ❖

Recipe texture: Very easy to chew if shrimp is finely chopped;
Soft and smooth if completely blended

1  8-ounce package fat-free cream
   cheese
2  tablespoons low-fat mayonnaise
1  12-ounce package extra-firm
   low-fat tofu
2  tablespoons lime juice
1  tablespoon soy sauce
¼  teaspoon garlic powder

¼  teaspoon ginger
¼  cup chopped sweet onion
2  tablespoons chopped parsley
   (optional)
½  pound shrimp, cooked, shelled,
   and deveined
salt and freshly ground pepper to
   taste

In a food processor, combine all ingredients except shrimp, salt, and
pepper. Blend until smooth. Add shrimp and process to desired consistency. Taste and adjust seasonings with salt and pepper to suit your
taste.

*Note:* The shrimp can remain in small pieces or be blended until
smooth. Sour cream (1½ cups) may be substituted for the tofu.

NUTRITIONAL INFORMATION PER SERVING

Calories 50; Fat 0.5 gm.; Protein 9 gm.; Carbohydrate 2 gm.;
Cholesterol 50 mg.; Fiber 0.1 gm. (very low)

# Roasted Red Pepper and Bean Dip

❖

*The wonderful flavor of this dip makes it a big hit as an appetizer. Serve as a spread on pita bread or as a dip for vegetables or soft tortilla pieces.*

❖ SERVES 10 ❖

Recipe texture: Very easy to chew;
Soft and smooth if completely blended

| | |
|---|---|
| 1 15-ounce can Great Northern beans, drained | ½ teaspoon cumin |
| | ¼ teaspoon garlic powder |
| 1 6-ounce package extra-firm tofu | ½ cup diced canned roasted red peppers |
| ⅓ cup fresh cilantro or parsley, chopped | dash Tabasco sauce to taste |
| 2 tablespoons lime juice | salt and freshly ground pepper to taste |
| 1 tablespoon olive oil | |

In a food processor, combine beans, tofu, cilantro, lime juice, olive oil, cumin, and garlic powder. Process until smooth. Stir in roasted peppers. Process briefly if desired. Add Tabasco, salt, and pepper to taste.

*Note:* Sour cream or fat-free sour cream (¾ cup) can be substituted for the tofu. However, the mixture will be thinner.

NUTRITIONAL INFORMATION PER SERVING

Calories 80; Fat 2 gm.; Protein 5 gm.; Carbohydrate 1 gm.; Cholesterol 0 mg.; Fiber 3 gm. (medium)

# *Salmon Log*

❖

*This is so good it could be served as a main course.*

❖ SERVES 6 ❖

Recipe texture: Very easy to chew

1  8-ounce package fat-free or low-fat cream cheese, room temperature
1  tablespoon fat-free mayonnaise
¼  cup chopped red onion
1  teaspoon horseradish

1  tablespoon lemon juice
⅛  teaspoon white pepper
1  15-ounce can salmon, drained
salt and freshly ground pepper to taste

In a food processor, combine cream cheese, mayonnaise, onion, horseradish, lemon juice, and pepper. Blend until well mixed. Set aside.

Remove and discard large bones and skin from canned salmon. Place salmon in medium bowl and combine with cream cheese mixture. Stir until well mixed. Add salt and pepper to taste, and extra horseradish, if desired. Form into 2 medium-sized logs or 1 round ball, or spoon into a serving bowl. Refrigerate until ready to serve.

*Note:* For a smoother consistency, add salmon to the cream cheese mixture in the food processor after removing bones and skin. Process until smooth.

NUTRITIONAL INFORMATION PER SERVING

Calories 125; Fat 4 gm.; Protein 20 gm.; Carbohydrate 2 gm.;
Cholesterol 50 mg.; Fiber 0.2 gm. (low)

# Salmon Mousse

........................................... ❖ ...........................................

*This very special recipe can be served either
as an appetizer or as a light entrée. It is a treat
for a luncheon or late evening supper.*

❖ SERVES 12 ❖

Recipe texture: Very easy to chew

1   15-ounce can red salmon,
    drained
1   envelope (7 grams) unflavored
    gelatin
¼   cup cold water
½   cup boiling water
½   cup low-fat mayonnaise

1   tablespoon lemon juice
2   tablespoons finely chopped onion
    dash Tabasco sauce
¼   teaspoon paprika
¼   teaspoon salt
1   teaspoon dried dill weed
½   cup whipping cream

Place a small bowl and the beaters of an electric mixer in refrigerator to chill.

Remove large bones and skin from salmon. Flake salmon into small pieces and set aside. In a small bowl, combine gelatin and cold water. Add boiling water and stir until gelatin dissolves. Cool for about 1 hour or until mixture reaches room temperature.

In a medium bowl, combine gelatin mixture, mayonnaise, lemon juice, onion, Tabasco, paprika, salt, and dill weed. Whisk to blend. Refrigerate for about 15 minutes or until mixture begins to thicken slightly. Fold in salmon.

In the chilled bowl, whip cream with chilled beaters until peaks form. Fold cream gently into the salmon mixture. Transfer to an attractive serving bowl or a decorative mold. Cover and chill for several hours. Serve on crackers, thinly sliced French baguette, or small pieces of toast as an appetizer.

*Note:* This may also be served on a plate lined with lettuce leaves.

NUTRITIONAL INFORMATION PER SERVING

Calories 100; Fat 6 gm.; Protein 9 gm.; Carbohydrate 3 gm.;
Cholesterol 30 mg.; Fiber 0 gm.

# Soups

❖

*Broccoli Bisque*

*Broccoli Cheese Soup*

*Butternut Squash Soup*

*Carrot Soup with Fresh Mint*

*Cauliflower Soup*

*Chicken and White Bean Soup*

*Chilled Guacamole Soup*

*Chilled Spinach and Tarragon Soup*

*Cream of Mushroom Soup with Brandy*

*Curried Vegetable Chowder*

*Egg Drop Soup*

*Homemade Vegetable Broth*

*Mexican Chili*

*Potato and Sausage Chowder*

*Potato Mushroom Soup*

Spicy Black Bean and Kielbasa Soup

Split Pea Soup

White Chili

White Gazpacho

Zucchini Soup

*Note:* Serve soups prepared to the desired consistency. Any soup can be puréed in a food processor, or processed with an immersion blender in a cooking pan, to achieve the best consistency. Soups can be thinned or thickened to meet your needs. To thin, use extra broth or water. To thicken, use instant potato flakes, mashed cooked vegetables, or cream of rice.

# Broccoli Bisque

❖

*A delightfully seasoned creamy soup.*

❖ SERVES 4 ❖

Recipe texture: Soft and smooth

| | |
|---|---|
| 1 medium potato, peeled and chopped | ½ cup fat-free half-and-half |
| 1 small onion, chopped | ⅛ teaspoon white pepper |
| 1 14-ounce can fat-free chicken broth | ⅛ teaspoon nutmeg |
| 2 cups broccoli florets | salt and freshly ground pepper to taste |
| | ½ cup fat-free sour cream |

In a medium saucepan, combine potato, onion, and broth. Bring to a boil. Reduce heat, cover, and simmer until vegetables are tender. Add broccoli and cook just until tender. Remove from heat. Using a food processor or a handheld immersion blender, process until smooth. Add half-and-half, white pepper, and nutmeg. Heat through, but do not boil. Add additional broth if soup is too thick. Add salt and pepper to taste. Top each individual serving with a dollop of sour cream.

NUTRITIONAL INFORMATION PER SERVING

Calories 190; Fat 0 gm.; Protein 8 gm.; Carbohydrate 40 gm.;
Cholesterol 5 mg.; Fiber 5 gm. (very high)

# Broccoli Cheese Soup

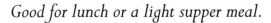

*Good for lunch or a light supper meal.*

❖ **S E R V E S  6** ❖

Recipe texture: Soft and smooth if completely blended

½  tablespoon canola oil
1  medium onion, finely chopped
2  large potatoes, peeled and cubed
½  teaspoon garlic powder
2  14-ounce cans fat-free chicken broth
1  bay leaf
4  cups chopped broccoli (about 1 pound)
1  cup shredded reduced-fat processed cheddar cheese
1  12-ounce can evaporated fat-free milk
¼  teaspoon white pepper
salt and freshly ground pepper to taste

Heat oil in a large heavy pot. Add onion and cook over medium heat until translucent. Add potatoes, garlic powder, 3 cups chicken broth, and bay leaf. Bring to a boil. Reduce heat, cover pan, and simmer for 20 to 30 minutes or until potatoes are tender.

Add broccoli and cook until tender. Discard bay leaf. Use an immersion blender to blend until smooth. Add cheese, milk, and white pepper. Heat gently until cheese has melted, but do not boil. Add salt and freshly ground pepper to taste. Add extra chicken broth if a thinner consistency is desired.

*Note:* If desired, remove part of the broccoli before blending. Return broccoli pieces to pan before serving. When reheating any leftover soup, do not bring it to a boil or the soup will curdle. It is fine to eat but not very attractive.

NUTRITIONAL INFORMATION PER SERVING
Calories 225; Fat 5 gm.; Protein 15 gm.; Carbohydrate 30 gm.;
Cholesterol 10 mg.; Fiber 4.2 gm. (very high)

# Butternut Squash Soup

······················· ❖ ·······················

*Squash never tasted so good!*

❖ SERVES 4 ❖

Recipe texture: Soft and smooth

3   pounds butternut squash
1   tablespoon olive oil
1   medium onion, diced
2   cloves garlic, minced
2   tablespoons minced cilantro
½   teaspoon curry powder
¼   teaspoon cumin
¼   teaspoon cinnamon
¼   teaspoon ground ginger

½   teaspoon dry mustard
¼   teaspoon white pepper
4   cups fat-free chicken broth,
    divided
½   cup orange juice
1   tablespoon lemon juice
salt to taste
½   cup fat-free sour cream

Preheat oven to 375 degrees. Cut squash in half lengthwise. (To make it easier to cut, microwave the squash for a few minutes before cutting.) Remove seeds and stringy fibers. Place cut-side down in a baking pan and add 1 inch of water to pan. Bake for 40 to 50 minutes or until soft.

While squash is baking, heat oil in a large soup pot. Add onion and cook until translucent. Add garlic, cilantro, curry powder, cumin, cinnamon, ginger, mustard, and white pepper. Mix well and cook 2 minutes. Set aside.

When squash is baked, scoop out pulp. There should be about 2 cups of squash. Place pulp and 1 cup of chicken broth in food processor. Blend until smooth. If necessary, strain to remove any stringy fibers. Add onion mixture to the food processor and blend with the squash. Return mixture to soup pot and add remaining 3 cups of chicken broth, orange juice, and lemon juice. Bring to a boil. Reduce heat and simmer for 20 to 40 minutes or until soup reaches desired consistency. Add extra broth if soup is too thick. Add salt to taste. Serve in heated soup bowls and top with a dollop of sour cream.

NUTRITIONAL INFORMATION PER SERVING

Calories 235; Fat 3 gm.; Protein 7 gm.; Carbohydrate 45 gm.;
Cholesterol 3 mg.; Fiber 5.9 gm. (very high)

# *Carrot Soup with Fresh Mint*

......................................... ❖ .........................................

*Loaded with vitamin A and beta carotene.*

❖ SERVES 6 ❖

Recipe texture: Soft and smooth

1  tablespoon butter or margarine
1  medium onion, chopped
2  pounds fresh carrots, peeled and
   chopped
¼  cup rice
6  cups fat-free chicken broth or
   vegetable broth
⅛  teaspoon white pepper

½  teaspoon ground ginger
6  fresh mint leaves
½  teaspoon sugar
salt and freshly ground pepper to
   taste
additional mint for garnish
   (optional)

Melt butter in a heavy medium soup pot. Add onion and cook over medium heat until translucent. Add carrots, rice, broth, white pepper, ginger, and mint. Bring to a boil. Reduce heat, cover, and simmer until carrots are tender.

Process soup until smooth in a food processor or with an immersion blender. Add additional broth if soup is too thick. Add sugar, salt, and freshly ground pepper to taste. Garnish with additional mint, if desired.

......................................................................................

NUTRITIONAL INFORMATION PER SERVING

Calories 120; Fat 2 gm.; Protein 3 gm.; Carbohydrate 23 gm.;
Cholesterol 5 mg.; Fiber 4.6 gm. (very high)

# Cauliflower Soup

❖

*Unusual, but so good.*

❖ SERVES 4 ❖

Recipe texture: Soft and smooth

1 pound cauliflower, chopped
1 medium potato, peeled and diced
1 small onion, chopped
1 15-ounce can Great Northern
  beans, drained
1 14-ounce can fat-free chicken
  broth

¼ teaspoon white pepper
1 cup fat-free half-and-half
½ cup fat-free milk, optional
salt and freshly ground pepper to
  taste

In a large soup pan, combine cauliflower, potato, onion, beans, and broth. Bring to a boil. Reduce heat, cover, and simmer until vegetables are tender, about 30 minutes.

In a food processor or with a handheld immersion blender, process soup to desired consistency. Add white pepper and half-and-half. Add milk if a thinner consistency is desired. Adjust seasoning with salt and pepper. Heat through.

NUTRITIONAL INFORMATION PER SERVING
Calories 250; Fat 0 gm.; Protein 14 gm.; Carbohydrate 48 gm.;
Cholesterol 2 mg.; Fiber 8 gm. (very high)

# Chicken and White Bean Soup

❖

*This mild flavored soup is a meal all its own.*

❖ SERVES 4 ❖

Recipe texture: Very easy to chew;
Soft and smooth if completely blended

| | |
|---|---|
| 1 tablespoon canola oil | 2 14-ounce cans fat-free chicken broth |
| 2 skinless, boneless chicken breasts, cubed | 1 15-ounce can Great Northern beans, drained |
| 1 medium onion, finely chopped | 1 bay leaf |
| ¼ teaspoon salt | ½ teaspoon thyme |
| ¼ teaspoon pepper | salt and freshly ground pepper to taste |
| 2 cloves garlic, minced | |
| 1 cup diced carrots | |

Heat oil in a medium soup pot. Add chicken and onion. Sprinkle with salt and pepper. Cook over medium heat until brown. Add garlic and carrots. Cook for 3 minutes. Add broth, beans, bay leaf, and thyme. Bring to a boil, reduce heat, and simmer until carrots are tender.

Remove bay leaf. Process soup to desired consistency. If soup is too thick, add extra broth. If soup is too thin, return to heat and simmer until soup is reduced. Add salt and pepper to taste.

NUTRITIONAL INFORMATION PER SERVING

Calories 260; Fat 5 gm.; Protein 28 gm.; Carbohydrate 26 gm.;
Cholesterol 50 mg.; Fiber 6.2 gm. (very high)

# Chilled Guacamole Soup

❖

*A light first-course soup.*

❖ SERVES 4 ❖

Recipe texture: Soft and smooth

2  14-ounce cans fat-free chicken broth
1  large avocado, peeled and chopped
1  cup fat-free sour cream, divided
1  small sweet onion, chopped
2  tablespoons lemon juice

2  cloves garlic, peeled and chopped
½  teaspoon chili powder
½  teaspoon cumin
salt and freshly ground pepper to taste
½  teaspoon paprika for garnish

In a food processor or blender, combine broth, avocado, ¾ cup sour cream, onion, lemon juice, garlic, chili powder, and cumin. Process until smooth. Add salt and pepper to taste. Add additional seasonings to taste if desired. Chill until ready to serve. Sprinkle each serving with paprika and top with a tablespoon of the remaining sour cream.

NUTRITIONAL INFORMATION PER SERVING

Calories 140; Fat 5 gm.; Protein 6 gm.; Carbohydrate 18 gm.;
Cholesterol 5 mg.; Fiber 1.8 gm. (medium)

# Chilled Spinach and Tarragon Soup

❖

*This elegant soup makes eating spinach easy.*

❖ SERVES 6 ❖

Recipe texture: Soft and smooth

| | |
|---|---|
| 2 tablespoons olive oil | 1 teaspoon dried tarragon |
| 1 large sweet onion, diced | 12 ounces fresh spinach, washed |
| 3 cloves garlic, minced | and stems removed |
| 4 cups fat-free chicken broth | 2 teaspoons Worcestershire sauce |
| 2 medium potatoes, peeled and | 1 teaspoon sugar |
| diced | Tabasco sauce, salt, and pepper to |
| ½ cup parsley, minced | taste |
| 1 tablespoon lemon juice | ½ cup fat-free sour cream |

Heat oil in a large heavy saucepan. Add onion and cook over medium heat until translucent. Add garlic and cook 2 minutes. Add chicken broth, potatoes, parsley, lemon juice, and tarragon. Bring to a boil, reduce heat, and simmer for 35 to 45 minutes, or until potatoes are tender.

Add spinach, cover, and cook 5 minutes, or until spinach is tender. Add Worcestershire sauce and sugar. Using an immersion blender or a food processor, process soup until smooth. Add additional chicken broth if soup is too thick. Add Tabasco, salt, and pepper to taste. Chill soup until ready to serve. Serve with a dollop of sour cream.

*Note:* This soup is also delicious served hot.

NUTRITIONAL INFORMATION PER SERVING

Calories 180; Fat 5 gm.; Protein 7 gm.; Carbohydrate 27 gm.;
Cholesterol 0 mg.; Fiber 3.5 gm. (high)

# Cream of Mushroom Soup with Brandy

❖

*The nutmeg and brandy will warm the heart.*

❖ SERVES 6 ❖

Recipe texture: Very easy to chew if partially blended;
Soft and smooth if blended until smooth

| | |
|---|---|
| 4 tablespoons butter or margarine | 3 cups fat-free milk |
| 1 large onion, chopped | ¼ teaspoon white pepper |
| 2 pounds fresh mushrooms, sliced | ¼ teaspoon nutmeg |
| 1 clove garlic, minced | 2 tablespoons brandy |
| 3 tablespoons flour | salt and freshly ground pepper to |
| 4 cups fat-free chicken broth | taste |

Melt butter in a large saucepan. Add onion, mushrooms, and garlic and cook until tender. Combine flour and part of the broth in a shaker. Shake until smooth. Add with the remaining broth to the pan. Stir constantly until mixture boils. Add milk, white pepper, and nutmeg. Use immersion blender and process until desired consistency. Stir in brandy just before serving. Add salt and pepper to taste.

NUTRITIONAL INFORMATION PER SERVING
Calories 175; Fat 8 gm.; Protein 9 gm.; Carbohydrate 17 gm.;
Cholesterol 25 mg.; Fiber 2 gm. (medium)

# *Curried Vegetable Chowder*

❖

*A good way to eat your vegetables.*

❖ SERVES 4 ❖

Recipe texture: Easy to chew;
Soft and smooth if blended

1　16-ounce package frozen
　cauliflower, broccoli, and carrot
　mix
1　cup fat-free chicken broth
1　cup evaporated fat-free milk
1　10¾-ounce can condensed cream
　of chicken soup

½　teaspoon curry powder
salt and freshly ground pepper to
　taste

In a large soup pan, combine all ingredients except salt and pepper. Bring to a boil, reduce heat, and simmer over very low heat for 20 minutes, or until vegetables are tender. (The soup will burn easily if pan gets too hot.) Use immersion blender and process soup to desired consistency. Add additional broth or milk if soup is too thick. Add salt and pepper to taste.

NUTRITIONAL INFORMATION PER SERVING
Calories 110; Fat 2 gm.; Protein 8 gm.; Carbohydrate 15 gm.;
Cholesterol 5 mg.; Fiber 2.8 gm. (medium)

# Egg Drop Soup

❖

*A light soup to whet the appetite.*

❖ SERVES 4 ❖

Recipe texture: Easy to chew if minced chicken is included;
Soft and smooth without the chicken or if soup is blended

| | |
|---|---|
| 6 cups fat-free chicken broth | 1 tablespoon white or rice vinegar |
| 3 tablespoons cornstarch | 2 eggs, lightly beaten |
| 3 tablespoons cold water | salt and pepper to taste |
| ½ teaspoon sugar | dash red pepper sauce (optional) |
| ⅛ teaspoon ground ginger | 2 scallions, chopped, for garnish |
| 1 tablespoon soy sauce | (optional) |

Bring chicken broth to a boil in a large saucepan. In a small dish, like a custard cup, mix cornstarch and water. Pour into broth, stirring constantly. Add sugar, ginger, soy sauce, and vinegar. While broth is actively boiling, pour beaten eggs into the broth, stirring slowly until the eggs separate in shreds. Remove from heat. Add salt, pepper, and red pepper sauce to taste. If soup is too thin, add additional cornstarch mixed with water to thicken to desired consistency. Garnish with scallions and serve.

*Note:* For extra protein, add cooked boneless minced chicken to the broth.

NUTRITIONAL INFORMATION PER SERVING
Calories 70; Fat 2 gm.; Protein 4 gm.; Carbohydrate 9 gm.;
Cholesterol 90 mg.; Fiber 0 gm.

# *Homemade Vegetable Broth*

❖

*Keep this on hand to thin soups and sauces.*

❖ SERVES 12 ❖

Recipe texture: Soft and smooth

3 cups chopped onion
2 cups chopped carrots
2 cups chopped celery
2 cups chopped parsnips
1 cup chopped leeks, white and
  light green parts
¼ cup lentils
4 cloves garlic

2 bay leaves
1 teaspoon basil
½ teaspoon thyme
½ teaspoon rosemary
8 whole peppercorns
5 quarts cold water
salt and freshly ground pepper to
  taste

In a large soup pot, combine all ingredients except salt and pepper.
Bring to a boil. Reduce heat and simmer for 1 to 2 hours. Pour mixture through strainer. Discard solids. Adjust seasoning with salt and pepper. Serve, and store remainder in the refrigerator or freezer.

NUTRITIONAL INFORMATION PER SERVING

Calories 20; Fat 0 gm.; Protein 0 gm.; Carbohydrate 5 gm.;
Cholesterol 0 mg.; Fiber low (if mixture is strained)

# Mexican Chili

❖

*This is a great chili recipe if you like your chili thick and flavorful. The refried beans in the recipe are the secret.*

❖ SERVES 6 ❖

Recipe texture: Easy to chew;
Soft and smooth if blended

| | | | |
|---|---|---|---|
| 1 | pound extra-lean ground beef | 1 | 15-ounce can kidney beans, |
| ½ | teaspoon salt | | undrained (optional) |
| ¼ | teaspoon pepper | 1½ | cups water |
| 1 | medium onion, finely chopped | 2 | teaspoons chili powder |
| 1 | 15-ounce can tomato sauce | 1 | teaspoon cumin |
| 1 | 15-ounce can refried beans | 1 | teaspoon molasses or sugar |

Brown meat in a large heavy saucepan, stirring as it cooks to break it up into small pieces. Sprinkle with salt and pepper. Add onion and cook until translucent. Drain off any excess fat and discard. Add all remaining ingredients. Bring to a boil. Reduce heat and simmer until flavors blend and chili reaches the desired consistency. Add extra water if needed. Check for seasoning and add extra chili powder or extra sweetness to taste.

*Note:* For a smoother consistency, use an immersion blender or food processor and process until smooth.

NUTRITIONAL INFORMATION PER SERVING
Calories 260; Fat 13 gm.; Protein 18 gm.; Carbohydrate 17 gm.;
Cholesterol 0 mg.; Fiber 4.0 gm. (high)

# Potato and Sausage Chowder

❖

*Hearty and full of flavor.*

❖ SERVES 8 ❖

Recipe texture: Easy to chew;
Soft and smooth if blended

½ pound low-fat Italian sausage,
  cut in small pieces
3 tablespoons butter or margarine
1 large onion, chopped
3 tablespoons flour
4 cups fat-free milk
3 medium potatoes, peeled and
  cubed (about 4 cups)

½ teaspoon salt
¼ teaspoon white pepper
8 ounces low-fat processed
  cheddar cheese, shredded
1 cup fat-free chicken broth
  (optional)
salt and freshly ground pepper to
  taste

In a medium skillet, cook sausage until brown. Remove sausage and set aside. Drain fat and discard. Melt butter in a large heavy saucepan. Add onion and cook over medium heat until translucent. Add flour and cook, stirring constantly until bubbly. Cook 2 minutes. Add milk and bring to a boil, stirring constantly. Add potatoes, salt, and pepper. Cover and simmer about 25 minutes or until potatoes are tender.

Stir in cheese and sausage. Heat through. Add chicken broth if a thinner soup is desired. Adjust seasonings to taste.

*Note:* For a smoother consistency, place soup in a food processor or use an immersion blender to process to desired consistency.

NUTRITIONAL INFORMATION PER SERVING

Calories 385; Fat 17 gm.; Protein 19 gm.; Carbohydrate 39 gm.;
Cholesterol 45 mg.; Fiber 2 gm. (medium)

# *Potato Mushroom Soup*

❖

*Flavorful herbs and white pepper
add just the right seasoning.*

❖ SERVES 6 ❖

Recipe texture: Very easy to chew;
Soft and smooth if blended

2 tablespoons butter or margarine
2 medium leeks chopped, white and light green parts
1 pound fresh mushrooms, sliced
2 large carrots, chopped
6 cups fat-free chicken broth
½ teaspoon dried Italian seasoning or dill weed
½ teaspoon white pepper
1 bay leaf
½ teaspoon salt
5 medium potatoes, peeled and diced
1 cup fat-free milk
2 tablespoons flour
salt and freshly ground pepper to taste
sprig of fresh herbs for garnish

Melt butter in a large stock pot. Add leeks and cook over medium heat for 3 to 4 minutes or until tender. Add mushrooms and cook until mushrooms are soft. Add carrots, chicken broth, Italian seasoning, white pepper, bay leaf, salt, and potatoes. Bring to a boil. Reduce heat and simmer for about 1 hour or until potatoes are very tender.

Mix milk and flour in a shaker. Pour into soup, stirring constantly. Bring to a boil and cook 2 minutes, until soup thickens

*(continued)*

## *Potato Mushroom Soup (continued)*

slightly. Remove bay leaf. If soup is too thin, add additional flour to thicken. If soup is too thick, add additional broth or milk. Add salt and pepper to taste. Garnish with a sprig of fresh herbs.

*Note:* For a smoother consistency, use immersion blender and blend to desired consistency.

NUTRITIONAL INFORMATION PER SERVING

Calories 165; Fat 4 gm.; Protein 7 gm.; Carbohydrate 25 gm.;
Cholesterol 10 mg.; Fiber 3 gm. (high)

# Spicy Black Bean and Kielbasa Soup

❖

*The kielbasa gives this soup a wonderful rich flavor.*

❖ SERVES 4 ❖

Recipe texture: Easy to chew if kielbasa is finely chopped;
Soft and smooth if blended

| | |
|---|---|
| 1 tablespoon olive oil | 1 teaspoon chili powder |
| 1 large onion, diced | ½ teaspoon cumin |
| 1 clove garlic, minced | ¼ teaspoon pepper |
| 2 15-ounce cans black beans, drained and rinsed | dash Tabasco sauce |
| 2 cups fat-free chicken broth | ¼ pound pre-cooked low-fat kielbasa, finely chopped |

Heat oil in a small skillet. Add onions and cook over medium heat until translucent. Add garlic and cook 1 minute. Spoon into a food processor. Add beans and broth. Process until smooth. Pour bean mixture into a medium saucepan. Add chili powder, cumin, pepper, and Tabasco. Bring to a boil, reduce heat, and simmer for 30 minutes. Add additional broth or water if soup is too thick. Add kielbasa to soup and heat through.

*Note:* If a smooth soup is desired, process kielbasa in a food processor with a small amount of broth before adding to the soup.

NUTRITIONAL INFORMATION PER SERVING
Calories 300; Fat 12 gm.; Protein 16 gm.; Carbohydrate 32 gm.;
Cholesterol 20 mg.; Fiber 12 gm. (very high)

# Split Pea Soup

........................................... ❖ ...........................................

*What a great meal to make ahead! Enjoy the aroma
as it cooks. Make an extra-large batch and
freeze leftovers in small containers.*

❖ SERVES 8 ❖

Recipe texture: Very easy to chew;
Soft and smooth if blended

| | | | |
|---|---|---|---|
| 1 | pound dry green split peas (2 cups) | 2 | garlic cloves, minced |
| 2 | 14-ounce cans chicken broth | 2 | large potatoes, peeled and diced |
| 4 | cups water | 4 | chicken bouillon cubes |
| 1 | tablespoon vegetable oil | ½ | teaspoon thyme |
| 1 | large onion, chopped | 1 | bay leaf |
| 3 | stalks celery, chopped | 1 | pound lean ham, diced |
| 2 | large carrots, peeled and chopped | | salt and freshly ground pepper to taste |
| 1 | small shallot, minced | | |

Wash peas in a colander. Place peas in large cooking pot and cover with water. Bring to a boil. Remove from heat and let set for 1 to 2 hours.

Drain off water. Add chicken broth and 4 cups water. Bring to a boil again. Reduce heat and simmer for 1 to 2 hours until peas are tender and mushy. Add additional water if needed. (Do not add any salt, salty foods, or high-acid foods before the peas are soft. Salt and acid will prevent the peas from becoming soft.)

While peas are cooking, heat oil in medium skillet. Add onion and cook until translucent. Add celery and carrots and cook until soft. Add shallot and garlic. Cook 1 minute. Remove from heat.

When peas are soft, add cooked vegetables, potatoes, bouillon cubes, thyme, bay leaf, and ham. Cook until potatoes are tender and soup has reached desired consistency. If soup is too thick, thin with water or chicken broth. Remove bay leaf before serving. Adjust seasoning with salt and pepper to taste.

*Note:* For a very smooth consistency, process soup in a food processor or blender.

NUTRITIONAL INFORMATION PER SERVING

Calories 370; Fat 5 gm.; Protein 30 gm.; Carbohydrate 52 gm.;
Cholesterol 25 mg.; Fiber 20 gm. (very high)

# White Chili

*Create this unique chili with cumin,*
*oregano, chicken, and white beans.*

❖ SERVES 6 ❖

Recipe texture: Easy to chew;
Soft and smooth if blended

| | | | |
|---|---|---|---|
| 1 | tablespoon olive oil | 4 | cups fat-free chicken broth |
| 1 | large onion, chopped | 1 | teaspoon cumin |
| 2 | boneless, skinless chicken breasts, cut in bite-size pieces | 2 | teaspoons oregano |
| 2 | cloves garlic, minced | | salt and freshly ground pepper to taste |
| 2 | 15-ounce cans navy beans or other white beans, drained | | dash cayenne pepper (optional) |
| | | 6 | tablespoons fat-free sour cream |

Heat oil in a large pan. Add onion and cook over medium heat until translucent. Add chicken and cook until brown. Add garlic and cook 1 minute. Add beans, chicken broth, cumin, and oregano. Bring to a boil, reduce heat, and simmer for 20 to 30 minutes. Add salt and pepper to taste. If a thinner consistency is desired, add extra broth. For a hotter chili, add cayenne pepper to suit your taste. Serve in warm bowls topped with a dollop of sour cream.

*Note:* For a smoother consistency, process until smooth in a food processor or with an immersion blender.

NUTRITIONAL INFORMATION PER SERVING
Calories 245; Fat 3 gm.; Protein 20 gm.; Carbohydrate 35 gm.;
Cholesterol 20 mg.; Fiber 7 gm. (very high)

# *White Gazpacho*

❖

*This is a refreshing cold soup to serve as a light first course.*

❖ SERVES 6 ❖

Recipe texture: Easy to chew if garnished;
Soft and smooth without garnish

3   medium cucumbers, peeled, seeded, and cubed
2   cloves garlic, minced
2   cups fat-free sour cream
1   cup fat-free plain yogurt
2   cups fat-free chicken broth or vegetable broth, divided

3   dashes Tabasco sauce
salt and freshly ground pepper to taste
½   cup chopped tomatoes (optional)
2   tablespoons chopped parsley (optional)

In a food processor, combine cucumbers, garlic, sour cream, and yogurt. Add 1 cup of broth. Season with Tabasco, salt, and pepper to taste. Place in covered bowl and refrigerate several hours or overnight. (The soup will thicken slightly.)

When ready to serve, thin with extra broth if desired. Top each serving with chopped tomatoes and parsley, if desired.

NUTRITIONAL INFORMATION PER SERVING
Calories 140; Fat 0 gm.; Protein 10 gm.; Carbohydrate 25 gm.;
Cholesterol 10 mg.; Fiber 2.6 gm. (medium)

# Zucchini Soup

❖

*A perfect summer soup when you have lots of fresh zucchini.*

❖ SERVES 4 ❖

Recipe texture: Very easy to chew if partially blended;
Soft and smooth if completely blended

| | |
|---|---|
| 1 tablespoon butter or margarine | 4 cups fat-free chicken broth |
| 1 medium onion, chopped | ¼ teaspoon white pepper |
| 2 pounds zucchini, peeled, seeds removed, and sliced (about 4 cups) | ½ cup shredded carrots |
| | ½ cup white wine |
| 2 medium potatoes, peeled and diced | salt and freshly ground pepper to taste |

Melt butter in a large saucepan. Add onion and cook over medium heat until translucent. Add zucchini, potatoes, chicken broth, and white pepper. Boil gently for 30 minutes or until vegetables are tender. Using an immersion blender, process until smooth. Add carrots and cook 10 minutes or until carrots are tender. Add wine and keep warm until ready to serve. Add additional broth if soup is too thick. Season with salt and pepper.

*Note:* For a smoother consistency, blend soup after the carrots have been added and process until smooth.

NUTRITIONAL INFORMATION PER SERVING
Calories 120; Fat 3 gm.; Protein 6 gm.; Carbohydrate 17 gm.;
Cholesterol 10 mg.; Fiber 4 gm. (high)

# MAIN COURSES

❖

*Beef Burgundy*

*Beef Stroganoff*

*Brandy Chicken Breasts*

*Chicken à la King*

*Chicken in Mushroom Sauce*

*Cinnamon-Apricot Glazed Salmon*

*Crab and Asparagus Linguine*

*Crab Cakes*

*Crab Imperial*

*Grilled Tuna with Avocado Butter*

*Halibut with Cilantro-Orange Sauce*

*Ham Loaf*

*Ham Strata*

*Hamburgers Extra Special*

*Lemon-Mustard Cod*

*Lobster Bisque*

*Meat Loaf*

*Pizza Popover Pie*

*Poor Man's Stroganoff*

## MAIN COURSES *(continued)*

*Pork and Squash Stew*

*Pork Tenderloin with Cinnamon Apples*

*Pork Tenderloin with Sherry-Mushroom Sauce*

*Salmon Loaf with Dill Sauce*

*Salmon with Dijon Wine Sauce*

*Saucy Chicken Casserole*

*Saucy Meatballs*

*Sausage and Grits Breakfast Casserole*

*Seafood Newburg*

*Sherried Beef Sirloin Tips*

*Shrimp and Mushroom Soufflé*

*Shrimp and Pasta Salad*

*Swordfish with Lemon-Lime Marinade*

*Tomato, Sausage, and Red Wine Pasta Sauce*

# *Beef Burgundy*

❖

*This is one of those times when canned soup in a recipe makes dinner so easy and yet so good. Your family will love it, and there will be enough left over for another meal. It is also a crowd pleaser for a large group of guests.*

❖ SERVES 10 ❖

Recipe texture: Easy to chew

1   tablespoon corn oil
2   large onions, sliced
3   pounds lean beef, cubed
1   teaspoon pepper
2   cloves garlic, minced
1   pound fresh mushrooms, sliced
1   cup Burgundy or other dry red
    wine

1   10¾-ounce can condensed cream
    of mushroom soup, undiluted
1   1-ounce package dry onion soup
    mix
1   10¾-ounce can beef consommé

Preheat oven to 325 degrees. Heat oil in a large heavy ovenproof pan or Dutch oven. Add onions and cook over medium heat until onions are translucent. Add beef and cook until brown, stirring occasionally. Add pepper, garlic, and mushrooms. Cook about 3 minutes, stirring occasionally, until mushrooms have softened. Add wine, mushroom soup, dry onion soup mix, and beef consommé. Cover pan. Bake for 1½ hours or until meat is tender and sauce has thickened. Check occasionally and add water if sauce gets too thick. Serve over cooked noodles.

NUTRITIONAL INFORMATION PER SERVING WITHOUT THE NOODLES

Calories 300; Fat 18 gm.; Protein 28 gm.; Carbohydrate 8 gm.;
Cholesterol 80 mg.; Fiber 1.3 gm. (medium)

# *Beef Stroganoff*

......................................... ❖ .........................................

*So tender and so flavorful.*

❖ SERVES 6 ❖

Recipe texture: Easy to chew;
Very easy to chew if meat is minced

3  tablespoons flour
¼  teaspoon salt
½  teaspoon pepper
1½ pounds beef tenderloin, cut in
   thin strips
2  tablespoons canola oil
½  pound fresh mushrooms, thickly
   sliced

1  14-ounce can fat-free beef broth
½  cup fat-free sour cream
2  tablespoons tomato paste
½  teaspoon paprika
salt to taste

Mix, flour, salt, and pepper in plastic bag. Add meat, seal bag, and shake until meat is coated. Heat oil in a heavy skillet. Add beef strips and cook until browned. Add mushrooms and cook until tender. Slowly add beef broth to skillet, stirring well to deglaze the pan. Bring to a boil. Reduce heat, cover, and simmer for 30 to 45 minutes or until meat is very tender. Add extra broth or water if needed.

In a small bowl, combine sour cream, tomato paste, and paprika. Slowly stir sour cream mixture into beef mixture. Turn heat to low and heat through. Do not boil. Add salt to taste. Serve over cooked noodles.

*Note:* If a less tender cut of meat is used, simmer 2 to 3 hours or until meat is very tender.

.........................................................................

NUTRITIONAL INFORMATION PER SERVING WITHOUT THE NOODLES

Calories 380; Fat 30 gm.; Protein 22 gm.; Carbohydrate 6 gm.;
Cholesterol 95 mg.; Fiber 0.4 gm. (low)

# *Brandy Chicken Breasts*

❖

*A wonderful flavor combination for a tender chicken dish.*

❖ SERVES 6 ❖

Recipe texture: Easy to chew

1 tablespoon canola oil
6 chicken breasts, skinned
¼ teaspoon garlic powder
½ teaspoon pepper
1 10¾-ounce can condensed cream of chicken soup

1 cup fat-free sour cream
¼ cup brandy
½ cup grated Parmesan cheese

Preheat oven to 350 degrees. Grease a 9 × 13-inch baking pan. Heat oil in a large skillet. Add chicken and brown over medium-high heat. (Chicken should be brown on the outside but does not need to be cooked through.) Place chicken in baking pan. Sprinkle chicken with garlic powder and pepper. In a small bowl, combine soup, sour cream, and brandy. Spoon over the chicken. Sprinkle with Parmesan cheese. Bake for 45 to 60 minutes. Check occasionally and add a little water if it gets too dry.

NUTRITIONAL INFORMATION PER SERVING

Calories 310; Fat 6 gm.; Protein 56 gm.; Carbohydrate 8 gm.;
Cholesterol 140 mg.; Fiber 0.5 gm. (low)

# Chicken à la King

············································· ❖ ·············································

*This is real comfort food. It looks so creamy and tastes wonderfully rich, but is deceivingly low in fat.*

❖ SERVES 6 ❖

Recipe texture: Easy to chew;
Very easy to chew if chicken and vegetables are minced;
Soft and smooth if blended

| | |
|---|---|
| 3 tablespoons butter or margarine | 1 cup low-fat chicken broth |
| 3 boned and skinned chicken breasts, cut in 1-inch pieces | 1 cup evaporated fat-free milk |
| 1 small onion, finely chopped | ¼ teaspoon white pepper |
| ½ pound fresh mushrooms, sliced | ¼ cup chopped parsley |
| 1 medium red pepper, diced | salt and freshly ground pepper to taste |
| ¼ cup flour | |

Melt butter in a large heavy saucepan. Add chicken and cook over medium heat until brown on the outside and completely done in the inside. Add onion and cook until translucent. Add mushrooms and red pepper. Cook until tender.

Combine flour and broth in a shaker. Add to pan with the evaporated milk. Bring to a boil, stirring constantly, until liquid thickens. Add additional broth if mixture is too thick, or additional flour mixed

with broth if it is too thin. Add white pepper and parsley. Adjust seasoning with salt and pepper.

Serve on toasted bread or noodles, or in puff pastry shells.

*Note:* If a smoother sauce is desired, use an immersion blender or a
food processor and process to the desired consistency.

........................................................................

NUTRITIONAL INFORMATION PER SERVING WITHOUT TOAST

Calories 200; Fat 7 gm.; Protein 18 gm.; Carbohydrate 16 gm.;
Cholesterol 45 mg.; Fiber 1.2 gm. (medium)

# Chicken in Mushroom Sauce

........................................ ❖ ........................................

*Super easy and super good.*

❖ SERVES 4 ❖

Recipe texture: Easy to chew;
Very easy to chew if chicken is cut or finely diced

| | | |
|---|---|---|
| 3 | tablespoons butter or margarine | ½ teaspoon salt |
| 4 | boned and skinned chicken breasts, thinly sliced | ½ teaspoon freshly ground black pepper |
| 1 | pound fresh mushrooms, sliced | ¼ teaspoon paprika |
| ½ | cup fat-free chicken broth | fresh tarragon or fresh parsley for garnish |
| 2 | tablespoons Dijon mustard | |
| 1 | teaspoon dried tarragon | |

Preheat oven to 350 degrees. Grease an 11 × 9-inch baking pan. Melt butter in a medium skillet. Add chicken and brown quickly over medium heat. (Chicken should not be cooked through at this point.) Remove chicken from skillet and place in baking pan. Add mushrooms to skillet and cook over medium heat until tender. Add chicken broth and stir to deglaze the pan. Remove from heat and stir in mustard, tarragon, salt, and pepper. Spoon mixture over chicken. Cover and bake 30 to 45 minutes or until chicken is very tender. Check occasionally and add extra broth or water if pan is getting too dry.

Serve chicken topped with sauce. Sprinkle with paprika and garnish with fresh tarragon or parsley.

....................................................................

NUTRITIONAL INFORMATION PER SERVING
Calories 190; Fat 10 gm.; Protein 23 gm.; Carbohydrate 8 gm.;
Cholesterol 75 mg.; Fiber 1.7 gm. (medium)

# Cinnamon-Apricot Glazed Salmon

❖

*The sweet apricot flavor complements the salmon.*

❖ SERVES 4 ❖

Recipe texture: Very easy to chew

| | |
|---|---|
| 2 tablespoons soy sauce | 12 ounces apricot nectar |
| ½ teaspoon ground ginger | 1½ pounds salmon fillet |
| 1 cinnamon stick | |

In a small saucepan, combine soy sauce, ginger, cinnamon stick, and apricot nectar. Bring to a boil, reduce heat, and boil gently until mixture is reduced to ¾ cup.

Preheat broiler. Remove skin from salmon. Place salmon fillets on broiler pan lined with foil. Broil for 5 minutes. Brush with apricot mixture. Continue to broil until lightly brown and completely done on one side. Turn carefully with a spatula, baste, and broil the other side.

NUTRITIONAL INFORMATION PER SERVING

Calories 260; Fat 6 gm.; Protein 35 gm.; Carbohydrate 16 gm.;
Cholesterol 90 mg.; Fiber 2.4 gm. (medium)

# Crab and Asparagus Linguine

❖

*A touch of elegance.*

❖ SERVES 4 ❖

Recipe texture: Easy to chew

12 ounces linguine or other pasta
1   10¾-ounce can condensed cream of chicken or cream of chicken with herbs soup
1   cup fat-free half-and-half
1   cup shredded low-fat mozzarella cheese

6   ounces crab meat, canned or frozen
¼   cup white wine
2   cups chopped fresh or frozen asparagus, blanched
½   cup chicken broth (optional)

**Topping**

½   cup seasoned bread crumbs
1   tablespoon butter or margarine, melted

¼   cup fat-free half-and-half
nonstick cooking spray

Preheat oven to 350 degrees. Butter an 8 × 8-inch baking pan or casserole dish. Cook linguine according to package directions until al dente. Drain and set aside.

While pasta is cooking, combine soup and half-and-half in a large bowl. Stir in cheese, crab, and wine. Add cooked linguine and asparagus. Toss gently to mix. Add chicken broth to thin if the mixture needs extra liquid. Spoon into prepared baking pan.

In a small bowl, combine bread crumbs, butter, and half-and-half. Stir until mixed. Sprinkle over linguine. Spray topping with nonstick cooking spray to coat well. Bake for 30 minutes or until top is golden brown and casserole is heated through.

This may be made ahead and refrigerated before baking. If baking when cold, add 15 to 20 minutes to the baking time.

*Note:* Green beans or broccoli may be substituted for the asparagus. Other cheese of your choice may be substituted for the mozzarella cheese.

······································································································

NUTRITIONAL INFORMATION PER SERVING INCLUDING THE PASTA

Calories 625; Fat 14 gm.; Protein 35 gm.; Carbohydrate 90 gm.;
Cholesterol 70 mg.; Fiber 2.3 gm. (medium)

# Crab Cakes

❖

*This special treat is very easy to make.*

❖ SERVES 4 ❖

Recipe texture: Very easy to chew

2   slices bread, crusts removed
2   tablespoons milk
1   tablespoon low-fat mayonnaise
1   teaspoon Dijon mustard
1   teaspoon Worcestershire sauce
1   teaspoon baking powder
¼   teaspoon salt

⅛   teaspoon pepper
1   teaspoon seafood seasoning (see note)
1   large egg, lightly beaten
1   pound crabmeat
1   tablespoon canola oil

Break bread into small pieces and place in large bowl. Add milk and stir to moisten. Add all remaining ingredients except canola oil. Mix thoroughly. Form into 4 to 6 cakes. Heat oil in nonstick skillet. Sauté cakes over medium-low heat for 5 minutes on each side or until lightly brown and done in the middle.

*Note:* Old Bay seasoning is one popular brand of seafood seasoning you may want to try. It is a mixture of celery salt, pepper, cloves, allspice, ginger, mace, cardamom, cinnamon, and paprika.

NUTRITIONAL INFORMATION PER SERVING
Calories 200; Fat 7 gm.; Protein 26 gm.; Carbohydrate 8 gm.;
Cholesterol 150 mg.; Fiber 0.3 gm. (low)

# *Crab Imperial*

............................... ❖ ...............................

*A meal for a special occasion.*

❖ SERVES 4 ❖

Recipe texture: Easy to chew;
Very easy to chew without the bell peppers

| | |
|---|---|
| 4 tablespoons butter or margarine | 2 egg yolks, lightly beaten |
| ⅓ cup flour | 1 teaspoon Worcestershire sauce |
| 2½ cups fat-free milk | dash Tabasco sauce |
| ¼ teaspoon white pepper | salt and freshly ground pepper to |
| ⅓ cup diced green bell pepper (optional) | taste |
| | 12 ounces crabmeat, canned or |
| ⅓ cup diced red bell pepper (optional) | frozen |
| | ½ cup grated Parmesan cheese |

Melt butter in a medium heavy saucepan. Add flour and cook for 2 minutes over medium heat, stirring constantly with a wooden spoon. Add milk, white pepper, and bell peppers. Bring to a boil, stirring constantly. Remove from heat. Place egg yolks in a custard cup. Add 2 tablespoons of the hot milk mixture to the egg yolks. Stir to warm the eggs. Add egg yolk mixture back to pan. Return pan to heat and cook until heated through, but do not boil. Add Worcestershire sauce and Tabasco. Add salt and pepper to taste. Add crab and stir gently.

Preheat broiler. Spoon crab mixture into small individual serving dishes or sea shells. Sprinkle with Parmesan cheese. Brown lightly under the broiler.

.......................................................................

NUTRITIONAL INFORMATION PER SERVING

Calories 340; Fat 18 gm.; Protein 27 gm.; Carbohydrate 17 gm.;
Cholesterol 215 mg.; Fiber 0.4 gm. (low)

# Grilled Tuna
# with Avocado Butter

❖

*This is so good, and healthy, too. Both the tuna and avocado are sources of good fats. The tuna has omega 3 fatty acids and the avocado is high in monounsaturated fat.*

❖ SERVES 4 ❖

Recipe texture: Easy to chew

| | |
|---|---|
| 1 large or 2 medium avocados, pitted and peeled | ½ tablespoon olive oil (optional) |
| | 2 teaspoons chili powder |
| 1 tablespoon butter or margarine, softened | 1 teaspoon cumin |
| | ¼ teaspoon salt |
| 1 tablespoon lime juice | dash garlic powder |
| ⅓ cup fresh cilantro, chopped | 1½ pounds tuna steak |

Heat grill to medium hot. In a food processor, combine avocado, butter, lime juice, and cilantro. Process until smooth. Add olive oil to thin, if desired. Spoon into a small bowl, cover tightly with plastic wrap, and refrigerate until ready to use. Combine chili powder, cumin, salt, and garlic powder. Rub mixture on tuna steaks. Place tuna on grill and cook for 10 to 15 minutes or until lightly brown and completely done in the middle. It should flake easily with a fork. Serve tuna with avocado butter.

*Note:* If you prefer milder seasoning, omit the chili powder and cumin. Sprinkle fish with salt, pepper, and any other seasonings of your choice.

NUTRITIONAL INFORMATION PER SERVING

Calories 330; Fat 17 gm.; Protein 40 gm.; Carbohydrate 4 gm.;
Cholesterol 70 mg.; Fiber 1.5 gm. (medium)

# Halibut with Cilantro-Orange Sauce

·································· ❖ ··································

*This is a mild fish with a flavorful sauce.*

❖ SERVES 4 ❖

Recipe texture: Easy to chew

2 pounds halibut fillet
1 tablespoon olive oil
1 medium sweet onion, diced
1 clove garlic, minced
¼ cup cilantro, minced
¼ teaspoon pepper
¼ teaspoon salt

1 cup orange juice
2 tablespoons fresh lemon juice
1 tablespoon lemon zest
1 tablespoon orange zest
½ tablespoon cornstarch
orange and lemon slices for garnish

Preheat oven to 400 degrees. Butter a 7 × 11-inch baking dish and place halibut fillets in it in one layer. Set aside.

Heat oil in a small skillet. Add onion and cook until translucent. Add garlic, cilantro, pepper, and salt. Cook 1 minute. Add orange juice, lemon juice, lemon zest, and orange zest. Mix and pour over fish. Loosely cover and bake for 20 to 30 minutes or until fish flakes when tested with a fork. Remove fish, place on a serving platter, and keep warm. Pour sauce into a small pan. In a small custard cup, mix cornstarch with 2 tablespoons cold water. Add to the pan and bring to a boil, stirring constantly until it thickens. If too thin, add extra cornstarch. If too thick, add extra orange juice. Pour over fish and garnish with lemon and orange slices.

·····················································································

NUTRITIONAL INFORMATION PER SERVING

Calories 315; Fat 8 gm.; Protein 49 gm.; Carbohydrate 12 gm.;
Cholesterol 75 mg.; Fiber 1.3 gm. (medium)

# Ham Loaf

❖

*Serve this for dinner and use the leftovers for sandwiches.*

❖ SERVES 6 ❖

Recipe texture: Easy to chew

| | |
|---|---|
| 1 pound ground lean ham | 1 tablespoon Dijon mustard |
| ½ pound ground lean pork | 1 tablespoon horseradish |
| 2 eggs, lightly beaten | 2 tablespoons onion, grated |
| ½ cup bread crumbs | ¼ teaspoon black pepper |
| ½ cup fat-free milk | ¼ teaspoon salt |
| ¼ cup brown sugar | |

**Topping**

¼ cup brown sugar                    2 teaspoons Dijon mustard

Preheat oven to 350 degrees. Grease a 9 × 5-inch loaf pan. In a large bowl, mix all ingredients except topping ingredients. Spoon into pan. Combine topping ingredients. Spread on top of ham mixture. Bake for 1 to 1½ hours or until a meat thermometer inserted in the middle reaches 165 degrees.

NUTRITIONAL INFORMATION PER SERVING

Calories 315; Fat 12 gm.; Protein 23 gm.; Carbohydrate 29 gm.;
Cholesterol 120 mg.; Fiber 0.6 gm. (low)

# *Ham Strata*

❖

*Make this ahead of time and
serve it later for brunch or supper.*

❖ SERVES 6 ❖

Recipe texture: Easy to chew

3   cups seasoned croutons
3   cups shredded low-fat cheddar
    cheese
6   eggs, lightly beaten
3   cups fat-free milk
1   small onion, minced

1   teaspoon dry mustard
½   teaspoon basil
¼   teaspoon thyme
¼   teaspoon marjoram
¾   pound ham, cubed or minced

Butter a 9 × 13-inch baking pan. Arrange croutons evenly in the pan.
Sprinkle with cheese. In a medium bowl, combine all remaining
ingredients. Pour over croutons and cheese. Cover and refrigerate
several hours or overnight. When ready to bake, preheat oven to 325
degrees. Bake for 1 hour or until set in the middle and lightly brown.
Let set for 10 minutes before cutting.

NUTRITIONAL INFORMATION PER SERVING
Calories 440; Fat 21 gm.; Protein 40 gm.; Carbohydrate 23 gm.;
Cholesterol 245 mg.; Fiber 1.2 gm. (medium)

# *Hamburgers Extra Special*

❖

*A soft hamburger that is so full of flavor.*

❖ SERVES 6 ❖

Recipe texture: Easy to chew

1 pound lean ground beef
1 cup (4 ounces) shredded low-fat
   cheddar cheese
1 egg, lightly beaten
2 or 3 medium tomatoes, peeled,
   seeded, and finely chopped

¼ cup finely chopped green olives
   (optional)
½ teaspoon onion powder
½ teaspoon salt
¼ teaspoon pepper

Combine all ingredients in a large bowl. Blend well. Shape into 4 patties. Place in nonstick skillet and cook over medium heat until completely done in the middle.

NUTRITIONAL INFORMATION PER SERVING

Calories 250; Fat 17 gm.; Protein 21 gm.; Carbohydrate 3 gm.;
Cholesterol 90 mg.; Fiber 0.7 gm. (low)

# Lemon-Mustard Cod

❖

*A lemon-mustard marinade and golden Parmesan topping
make this a truly enjoyable fish dish. And it is so easy!*

❖ SERVES 4 ❖

Recipe texture: Very easy to chew

1½ pounds cod fillets
½ teaspoon salt
¼ teaspoon pepper

2 tablespoons lemon juice
1 tablespoon Dijon mustard

**Topping:**
1 tablespoon butter or margarine,
  melted
2 tablespoons low-fat mayonnaise
½ teaspoon dry mustard

½ teaspoon dill weed
¼ cup grated Parmesan cheese
¼ teaspoon paprika
1 medium lemon, cut in thin slices

Grease broiler pan. Place fish on pan. Sprinkle with salt and pepper.

In a small bowl, combine lemon juice and Dijon mustard. Brush
on fish and let stand for 15 to 20 minutes. Preheat broiler.

In another small bowl, combine butter, mayonnaise, dry mustard,
dill weed, and Parmesan cheese. Set aside. Place fish 4 inches from
broiler and broil for about 5 minutes per side or until fish is almost
done. Spread mayonnaise mixture on top of fish and broil for 2 to 5
minutes more or until the topping is golden brown. Sprinkle with
paprika and garnish with lemon slices.

*Note:* Other firm fish, such as haddock, halibut, or salmon, may be
used.

NUTRITIONAL INFORMATION PER SERVING
Calories 190; Fat 6 gm.; Protein 26 gm.; Carbohydrate 6 gm.;
Cholesterol 15 mg.; Fiber 0.4 gm. (low)

# Lobster Bisque

❖

*Elegant but simple.*

❖ SERVES 6 ❖

Recipe texture: Very easy to chew;
Soft and smooth if blended

1½ pounds cooked lobster meat
4 tablespoons butter or margarine
1 medium onion, finely chopped
½ cup flour
2 14-ounce cans fat-free chicken broth

3 cups fat-free half-and-half
¾ cup dry sherry
1 tablespoon tomato paste
salt and freshly ground pepper to taste
½ cup chopped chives

Pick over lobster and discard any pieces of shell. Set aside. Melt butter in a large heavy saucepan. Add onion and cook over medium heat until translucent. Add flour and cook, stirring constantly, over medium heat for 2 minutes. Add chicken broth. Bring to a boil, stirring constantly. Boil gently for 3 minutes. Add half-and-half, sherry, and tomato paste. Add lobster and heat through. Add additional broth if soup is too thick. Garnish each bowl with a sprinkling of chives.

*Note:* For a smoother soup, use an immersion blender or a food processor to process to desired consistency.

NUTRITIONAL INFORMATION PER SERVING
Calories 325; Fat 9 gm.; Protein 25 gm.; Carbohydrate 29 gm.;
Cholesterol 100 mg.; Fiber 0.9 gm. (low)

# Meat Loaf

❖

*This is a simple, moist meat loaf. For a tomato flavor,*
*substitute tomato sauce for the milk.*
*Add seasonings of your choice.*

❖ SERVES 8 ❖

Recipe texture: Very easy to chew

1½ pounds lean ground beef
⅔ cup bread crumbs
¼ cup milk
2 eggs, lightly beaten

½ cup applesauce
1 teaspoon salt
1 teaspoon pepper

**Topping**
½ cup ketchup
1 tablespoon Worcestershire sauce

1 tablespoon Dijon mustard

Preheat oven to 350 degrees. Grease a 9 × 5-inch loaf pan. In a large mixing bowl, combine all ingredients except topping ingredients. Blend well. Spoon into loaf pan. In a small bowl, mix ketchup with Worcestershire sauce and mustard. Spread sauce on top of meat. Bake at 350 for 1 hour.

NUTRITIONAL INFORMATION PER SERVING
Calories 300; Fat 19 gm.; Protein 18 gm.; Carbohydrate 15 gm.;
Cholesterol 110 mg.; Fiber 1 gm. (medium)

# Pizza Popover Pie

❖

*A pizza-filled puff topped with cheese.*

❖ SERVES 6 ❖

Recipe texture: Easy to chew;
Soft and smooth if blended

| | |
|---|---|
| 1½ pounds extra lean ground beef | 2 cups (8 ounces) shredded mozzarella cheese |
| 1 15-ounce can tomato sauce | |
| 1 teaspoon Italian seasoning | 1 cup flour |
| ½ teaspoon garlic powder | 1 cup fat-free milk |
| ½ teaspoon onion powder | 2 eggs, lightly beaten |
| salt and pepper to taste | ⅓ cup grated Parmesan cheese |

Preheat oven to 375 degrees. Grease a shallow 2-quart casserole dish. In a medium skillet, brown ground beef over medium heat. Drain off and discard any fat. To the skillet, add tomato sauce, Italian seasoning, garlic powder, and onion powder. Bring to a boil and simmer for 10 minutes. Add salt and pepper to taste. Spoon into casserole. Sprinkle with mozzarella cheese. In a small bowl, combine flour, milk, and eggs. Mix well. Pour into casserole. Top with Parmesan cheese. Bake for 25 to 35 minutes or until the middle is set and the top is lightly browned.

*Note:* For a smoother consistency, place meat and tomato mixture in a food processor and blend until smooth before spooning into casserole.

NUTRITIONAL INFORMATION PER SERVING

Calories 485; Fat 25 gm.; Protein 40 gm.; Carbohydrate 25 gm.;
Cholesterol 165 mg.; Fiber 1.6 gm. (medium)

# Poor Man's Stroganoff

❖

*So easy and so good.*

❖ SERVES 6 ❖

Recipe texture: Easy to chew

1¼ pounds lean ground beef
½ teaspoon salt
½ teaspoon pepper
1 small onion, finely chopped
1 clove garlic, minced
½ pound fresh mushrooms, sliced
2 tablespoons flour

2 cups water or chicken broth, divided
1 10¾-ounce can condensed cream of chicken soup
1 cup fat-free sour cream

In a large nonstick skillet, brown beef over medium-high heat. Sprinkle with salt and pepper. Add onion and cook until tender. Add garlic and mushrooms and cook until mushrooms are tender. In a shaker, mix flour and ½ cup water (or broth, if using). Pour into skillet. Add remaining water and soup. Stir to mix. Bring to a boil, stirring constantly until mixture thickens. Add extra water or broth if sauce is too thick. Simmer for 15 to 30 minutes. Stir in sour cream and heat through. Serve with noodles or mashed potatoes.

NUTRITIONAL INFORMATION PER SERVING WITHOUT NOODLES
Calories 300; Fat 14 gm.; Protein 30 gm.; Carbohydrate 13 gm.;
Cholesterol 80 mg.; Fiber 0.9 gm. (low)

# Pork and Squash Stew

······························· ❖ ·······························

*This is a comfort food dish that smells and tastes wonderful.*

❖ SERVES 4 ❖

Recipe texture: Easy to chew;
Soft and smooth if blended in a food processor

| | | | |
|---|---|---|---|
| 1 | pound pork tenderloin, cut in ¾-inch cubes | 1 | cup sliced carrots |
| 3 | tablespoons flour | ½ | cup water or chicken broth |
| ½ | teaspoon salt | ½ | teaspoon crushed rosemary |
| ¼ | teaspoon pepper | 1½ | cups light beer |
| 2 | tablespoons canola oil, divided | 2 | cups cubed winter squash |
| 1 | large onion, chopped | | salt and freshly ground pepper to taste |

Combine pork, flour, salt, and pepper in a plastic bag. Seal bag and shake to coat meat. In a large nonstick skillet or Dutch oven, heat 1 tablespoon oil. Remove pork from bag and place in pan. Cook over medium to high heat until brown on all sides. Remove pork from skillet and set aside. Add the remaining 1 tablespoon oil, onion and carrots to the skillet. Cook until onions are translucent. Add water or broth to deglaze the pan. Return pork to skillet. Add rosemary, beer, and squash. Cover and simmer 30 minutes or until squash is tender. Add salt and pepper to taste. Check occasionally and add extra water or broth if needed. When ready to serve, ladle into bowls.

······························································

NUTRITIONAL INFORMATION PER SERVING

Calories 265; Fat 11 gm.; Protein 26 gm.; Carbohydrate 15 gm.;
Cholesterol 75 mg.; Fiber 2.2 gm. (medium)

# Pork Tenderloin with Cinnamon Apples

❖

*Use pork tenderloin for an extra tender meat dish.
Combined with fresh apples, cinnamon and
brown sugar, it is very special.*

❖ SERVES 4 ❖

Recipe texture: Easy to chew

| | |
|---|---|
| 1½ pounds pork tenderloin | ¼ cup orange juice |
| ½ teaspoon salt | ¼ cup dry sherry |
| ½ teaspoon pepper | ¼ cup brown sugar |
| 1 tablespoon canola oil | ¼ teaspoon cinnamon |
| 4 small apples, peeled and thickly sliced | ½ cup chicken broth (optional) |

Preheat oven to 350 degrees. Remove fat and white membrane from the tenderloin and cut it into ½-inch-thick slices. Sprinkle with salt and pepper. Heat oil in a large oven-proof skillet. Add pork and brown quickly over high heat. Remove skillet from heat. Arrange apples slices around the pan. Mix orange juice, sherry, brown sugar, and cinnamon. Pour over the pork and apples. Cover and bake 30 minutes. Uncover and bake another 20 minutes. Add broth or water if pan gets too dry.

*Note:* Pears, peaches, or apricots may be substituted for the apples.

NUTRITIONAL INFORMATION PER SERVING

Calories 425; Fat 13 gm.; Protein 49 gm.; Carbohydrate 29 gm.;
Cholesterol 120 mg.; Fiber 2.6 gm. (medium)

# Pork Tenderloin with Sherry-Mushroom Sauce

❖

*This wonderful family dish is great for company, too.*

❖ SERVES 4 ❖

Recipe texture: Easy to chew;
Very easy to chew if sauce is blended and meat is minced;
Soft and smooth if both meat and sauce are blended

| | |
|---|---|
| 1½ pounds pork tenderloin | 1    14-ounce can fat-free chicken broth |
| 2    tablespoons butter or margarine, divided | ¼    cup dry sherry |
| ½    teaspoon salt | ¼    teaspoon white pepper |
| ¼    teaspoon pepper | ¼    teaspoon ground thyme |
| 1    medium onion, thinly sliced | salt and freshly ground pepper to taste |
| 1    pound fresh mushrooms, sliced | |
| 3    tablespoons cornstarch | ½    cup fat-free sour cream |

Remove any fat and white membrane from pork tenderloin and cut it into ½-inch-thick slices. Melt 1 tablespoon butter in a large skillet. Add meat and cook over medium-high heat until brown on all sides. Sprinkle with salt and pepper. Remove from pan. Set aside and keep warm.

Add the remaining 1 tablespoon butter to skillet. Add onions and cook until onions are translucent. Push aside and add mushrooms. Cook until soft, stirring occasionally. Mix cornstarch with chicken broth and pour into skillet. Cook, stirring constantly, until mixture comes to a boil. Add sherry, white pepper, and thyme. Return meat to the skillet. Reduce heat and simmer over low heat until ready to serve. Add additional broth if sauce is too thick. Add salt and pepper to taste. When ready to serve, add sour cream. Heat through but do not boil. Arrange meat on a platter or on individual plates. Top with mushroom sauce.

*Note:* For a smoother sauce, place sauce in a food processor and blend until smooth.

NUTRITIONAL INFORMATION PER SERVING

Calories 350; Fat 12 gm.; Protein 41 gm.; Carbohydrate 19 gm.; Cholesterol 120 mg.; Fiber 2.1 gm. (medium)

# Salmon Loaf with Dill Sauce

················· ❖ ·················

*This old-time favorite is traditionally
served with creamed peas.*

❖ SERVES 6 ❖

Recipe texture: Very easy to chew

1   15-ounce can salmon, drained
2   eggs, lightly beaten
1½ cups dry bread crumbs

1   10¾-ounce can condensed
cream of celery soup

**Dill Sauce**

½   cup low fat mayonnaise
¼   cup fat-free sour cream
1   tablespoon lemon juice

½   teaspoon dill weed
dash white pepper
salt to taste

Preheat oven to 350 degrees. Grease a 7½ × 3¾-inch loaf pan.
Remove large bones and any black skin from the salmon. In a
medium bowl, combine salmon, eggs, bread crumbs, and soup. Stir
gently to mix. Spoon into pan. Bake for 50 to 60 minutes or until set.
Meanwhile, prepare dill sauce. In a small bowl, combine all sauce
ingredients. Serve with salmon loaf.

*Note:* This loaf cannot be cut into slices that stay together. It has a
very soft texture. Instead, use a wide spatula to spoon out individual
servings.

·······························································

NUTRITIONAL INFORMATION PER SERVING

Calories 285; Fat 9 gm.; Protein 21 gm.; Carbohydrate 30 gm.;
Cholesterol 100 mg.; Fiber 1.5 gm. (medium)

# Salmon with
# Dijon Wine Sauce

❖

*Salmon is high in the healthy omega 3 fats.*

❖ SERVES 4 ❖

Recipe texture: Easy to chew

| | |
|---|---|
| 2 tablespoons butter or margarine, melted | ¼ teaspoon pepper |
| 1 tablespoon olive oil | ⅓ cup white wine |
| 2 pounds salmon fillets | ¼ teaspoon dill weed or tarragon |
| ¼ teaspoon salt | 2 tablespoons Dijon-style mustard |
| | 1½ teaspoons butter |

Preheat oven to 400 degrees. Put the 2 tablespoons butter and the olive oil in a 9 × 12-inch baking dish or a dish that fits the fillets. Place fish in pan skin-side down. Sprinkle with salt and pepper. Turn fish and bake skin-side up for 10 minutes. Turn fish and bake for another 10 minutes or until fish is completely done and flakes easily with a fork.

While fish is baking, combine wine, dill weed, and mustard in a small saucepan. Heat over low heat. Remove from heat until fish is ready to serve. Reheat sauce, adding 1½ teaspoons butter. Top fish with sauce.

NUTRITIONAL INFORMATION PER SERVING

Calories 330; Fat 16 gm.; Protein 45 gm.; Carbohydrate 1 gm.;
Cholesterol 135 mg.; Fiber 0 gm.

# Saucy Chicken Casserole

........................................... ❖ ...........................................

*The aroma of this dish baking in the oven is irresistible.*

❖ SERVES 6 ❖

Recipe texture: Easy to chew;
Soft and smooth if blended in a food processor

| | |
|---|---|
| 6 boned and skinned chicken breast halves | 1 cup fat-free sour cream |
| 1 10¾-ounce can condensed cream of chicken soup | ¾ cup fat-free chicken broth |
| 1 10¾-ounce can condensed cream of mushroom soup | ½ teaspoon onion powder |
| | ½ teaspoon poultry seasoning |
| | ¼ teaspoon pepper |
| | ¼ teaspoon paprika |

Preheat oven to 325 degrees. Grease a 9 × 13-inch baking pan. Arrange chicken pieces in pan. In a medium bowl, combine chicken soup, mushroom soup, sour cream, chicken broth, onion powder, poultry seasoning, and pepper. Mix well. Pour over chicken. Sprinkle with paprika. Bake, uncovered, for 1 hour or until chicken is tender. Check occasionally and add extra broth or water if pan gets too dry.

.............................................................................

NUTRITIONAL INFORMATION PER SERVING
Calories 215; Fat 7 gm.; Protein 24 gm.; Carbohydrate 14 gm.;
Cholesterol 60 mg.; Fiber 0.3 gm. (low)

# *Saucy Meatballs*

❖

*Meatballs made special with a memorable sauce.*

❖ SERVES 8 ❖
Recipe texture: Very easy to chew;
Soft and smooth if blended in a food processor

1½ cups lean ground beef
1   cup dry bread crumbs
1   egg, lightly beaten

½   teaspoon onion powder
1   teaspoon salt
¼   teaspoon pepper

**Sauce**
½   cup catsup
2   tablespoons brown sugar
1   tablespoon lemon juice

1   16-ounce can cranberry sauce
1   12-ounce bottle chili sauce

Preheat oven to 300 degrees. In a large bowl, combine ground beef, bread crumbs, egg, onion powder, salt, and pepper. Stir to mix. Form into 30 small balls. Place in large casserole dish that has a cover. In a small bowl, combine catsup, brown sugar, lemon juice, cranberry sauce, and chili sauce. Pour over meatballs. Cover and bake for 1 to 2 hours or until completely done. (Meat should be cooked until brown in the middle without any pink color.) If desired, serve over cooked noodles.

*Note:* This dish can also be cooked in a slow cooker for 6 to 8 hours.

NUTRITIONAL INFORMATION PER SERVING WITHOUT NOODLES
Calories 325; Fat 9 gm.; Protein 11 gm.; Carbohydrate 50 gm.;
Cholesterol 50 mg.; Fiber 2.3 gm. (medium)

# Sausage and Grits
# Breakfast Casserole

............................... ❖ ...............................

*This sausage, cheese, and egg dish bound together by grits*
*is a popular Southern breakfast treat.*

❖ SERVES 6 ❖

Recipe texture: Easy to chew

½  pound lean bulk pork sausage
½  pound lean ground beef
1   cup grits
1   tablespoon butter or margarine
4   eggs, lightly beaten

⅓  cup fat-free milk
½  teaspoon salt
2   cups (8 ounces) shredded low-fat
    cheddar cheese, divided

Preheat oven to 350 degrees. Grease a 2-quart baking dish. In a
medium skillet, brown pork sausage and ground beef. Crumble any
large pieces of sausage. Drain off any fat and discard. Spoon meat
into baking dish and set aside.

In a small saucepan, cook grits according to package directions.
Stir in butter, eggs, milk, salt, and 1½ cups of the cheese. Mix well.
Pour over meat. Bake for 40 to 45 minutes or until the middle is set.
Top with remaining ½ cup of cheese and continue baking 3 to 5 min-
utes or just until cheese is melted. Let stand 10 to 15 minutes before
serving.

.............................................................

NUTRITIONAL INFORMATION PER SERVING

Calories 435; Fat 24 gm.; Protein 32 gm.; Carbohydrate 23 gm.;
Cholesterol 200 mg.; Fiber 3.1 gm. (medium)

# Seafood Newburg

......................... ❖ .........................

*This low-fat version of the
classic creamy Newburg is just as good.*

❖ SERVES 4 ❖

Recipe texture: Easy to chew;
Very easy to chew if seafood is finely chopped;
Soft and smooth if blended in a food processor

| | |
|---|---|
| 3 tablespoons butter or margarine | 1 cup cooked shrimp, lobster, crab, or firm fish |
| 2 tablespoons flour | |
| 1 cup fat-free half-and-half | salt and freshly ground pepper to taste |
| ½ cup fat-free milk | |
| 3 egg yolks, lightly beaten | ¼ teaspoon paprika |
| ¼ cup dry white wine | parsley for garnish |
| 1 teaspoon lemon juice | |

Melt butter in a medium skillet. Add flour and cook for 3 minutes over medium heat, stirring constantly. Add half-and-half and milk. Bring to a boil, stirring constantly. Remove from heat. Place beaten egg yolks in a small bowl. Add 1 tablespoon of the hot milk mixture to eggs and stir. Continue adding hot mixture, 1 tablespoon at a time, until egg mixture is warm. Pour egg mixture into pan and return to heat. Cook and stir until thickened, but do not boil. Add wine, lemon juice, and seafood. Heat through. Add additional milk if mixture is too thick. Adjust seasonings with salt and pepper. Serve in pastry shells or over rice or pasta. Sprinkle with paprika. Garnish with parsley.

......................................................

NUTRITIONAL INFORMATION PER SERVING WITHOUT NOODLES OR RICE

Calories 240; Fat 13 gm.; Protein 18 gm.; Carbohydrate 13 gm.;
Cholesterol 300 mg.; Fiber 0 gm.

# Sherried Beef Sirloin Tips

❖

*The flavor of this dish can't be beat and it is
so easy—put it in the oven and forget about it!
Make extra, because leftovers warm up beautifully.*

❖ SERVES 6 ❖

Recipe texture: Easy to chew;
Very easy to chew if meat is finely diced

2 pounds lean beef sirloin, cut in 1-inch cubes

1 10¾-ounce can condensed cream of mushroom soup

1 1⅜-ounce package dry onion soup mix

1 pound fresh mushrooms, thickly sliced

2 cups water

½ cup dry sherry

½ cup fat-free sour cream

Preheat oven to 325 degrees. In a large heavy pan or 1½-quart casserole, combine all ingredients except sour cream. Mix well. Cover tightly and bake for 2 to 3 hours or until meat is very tender. Turn oven down to 300 degrees after the first hour. Check occasionally and add additional water if it becomes too dry. Add sour cream right before serving and heat through. Serve over cooked noodles.

*Note*: There is no need to brown the meat for this recipe. Adjust the oven temperature to keep the mixture simmering gently.

NUTRITIONAL INFORMATION PER SERVING WITHOUT NOODLES

Calories 285; Fat 9 gm.; Protein 36 gm.; Carbohydrate 15 gm.;
Cholesterol 90 mg.; Fiber 1.6 gm. (medium)

# Shrimp and Mushroom Soufflé

❖

*This dish can be prepared in advance and baked when you need it.*

❖ SERVES 8 ❖

Recipe texture: Easy to chew;
Very easy to chew if shrimp and mushrooms are finely chopped

8   bread slices, cubed
2   cups small cooked shrimp, canned or frozen
1   8-ounce can mushrooms, drained and chopped
8   ounces low-fat shredded cheddar cheese

2   cups fat-free milk
3   eggs
½   teaspoon salt
¼   teaspoon pepper
½   teaspoon dry mustard
½   teaspoon paprika

Preheat oven to 325 degrees. Butter a 9 × 13-inch baking pan. Layer bread cubes, shrimp, mushrooms, and cheese in pan. In a medium bowl, combine milk, eggs, salt, pepper, and dry mustard. Beat until well mixed. Pour into pan. Bake uncovered for 50 to 70 minutes or until the middle is set and top is lightly browned. Let set 15 minutes before serving.

*Note:* If desired, mixture can be prepared ahead of time and baked later. Cover pan and refrigerate a few hours or overnight until ready to bake.

NUTRITIONAL INFORMATION PER SERVING
Calories 250; Fat 8 gm.; Protein 28 gm.; Carbohydrate 17 gm.;
Cholesterol 200 mg.; Fiber 0.9 gm. (low)

# *Shrimp and Pasta Salad*

❖

*This is a great, low-fat, healthy, and attractive luncheon salad. The old recipes used regular mayonnaise, which added hundreds of calories. Low-fat mayonnaise works well if creatively seasoned.*

❖ SERVES 6 ❖

Recipe texture: Easy to chew

6  ounces small pasta shells (2 cups)
½  cup finely chopped red onion

½  medium red pepper, finely diced
1  cup cooked peas
1  pound cooked shrimp

**Dressing**

½  cup low-fat mayonnaise
¼  cup fat-free sour cream
1  tablespoon lemon juice
1  teaspoon sugar

⅛  teaspoon dill weed
⅛  teaspoon tarragon
salt and freshly ground pepper to taste

**Alternate dressing**

⅔  cup low-fat or fat-free mayonnaise
2  tablespoons bottled French dressing

2  teaspoons lemon juice
salt and freshly ground pepper to taste

In a large saucepan, cook pasta in boiling salted water just until al dente. Pour into colander, chill under cold running water, and drain well. In a large bowl, combine pasta, onion, red pepper, peas, and shrimp. In a small bowl, combine dressing ingredients and mix well. Mix dressing with shrimp and pasta. Add salt and pepper to taste.

*Note:* Crab or surmi can be substituted for the shrimp. Add other vegetables as desired.

NUTRITIONAL INFORMATION PER SERVING

Calories 215; Fat 2 gm.; Protein 20 gm.; Carbohydrate 30 gm.;
Cholesterol 116 mg.; Fiber 1.2 gm. (medium)

# Swordfish with Lemon-Lime Marinade

❖

*The combination of flavors in this marinade complements the mild swordfish.*

❖ SERVES 4 ❖

Recipe texture: Easy to chew

| | |
|---|---|
| 2 pounds swordfish steaks | 1 tablespoon Dijon mustard |
| 2 tablespoons lemon juice | ¼ cup vegetable oil |
| 2 tablespoons lime juice | 2 teaspoons dill weed |
| 2 tablespoons soy sauce | ¼ teaspoon cayenne pepper |
| 2 tablespoons honey | ½ teaspoon salt |

Cut swordfish into 4 pieces. Place in resealable plastic bag. In a small jar, combine lemon juice, lime juice, soy sauce, honey, mustard, oil, dill weed, cayenne, and salt. Mix well and pour into bag with swordfish. Reseal and refrigerate several hours. When ready to serve, heat grill to medium-hot. Remove fish from bag and grill until lightly browned on both sides and fish flakes easily.

*Note:* Instead of grilling, the swordfish can be fried in a small amount of oil in a nonstick skillet. Fry over medium heat. Watch carefully to prevent burning.

NUTRITIONAL INFORMATION PER SERVING

Calories 315; Fat 12 gm.; Protein 45 gm.; Carbohydrate 6 gm.;
Cholesterol 90 mg.; Fiber 0.3 gm. (low)

# *Tomato, Sausage, and Red Wine Pasta Sauce*

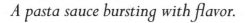

*A pasta sauce bursting with flavor.*

❖ SERVES 4 ❖

Recipe texture: Very easy to chew;
Soft and smooth if blended

| | |
|---|---|
| 1 tablespoon olive oil | ¼ cup vodka |
| 1 large onion, finely chopped | 2 14-ounce cans garlic-seasoned |
| 2 cloves garlic, minced | diced tomatoes |
| 6 ounces ground low-fat Italian | ½ cup fat-free half-and-half |
| sausage or ground beef | 1 teaspoon sugar, or to taste |
| 1 teaspoon ground fennel seed | salt and freshly ground pepper to |
| (optional) | taste |
| ½ cup dry red wine | |

Heat oil in a medium saucepan or large skillet. Add onion and cook over medium heat until translucent. Add garlic and cook 1 minute. Add sausage and cook until browned. Drain and discard fat. Add fennel, wine, vodka, and tomatoes. Bring to a boil, reduce heat and simmer for 20 to 30 minutes. Add half-and-half and heat through. Add sugar, salt, and pepper to taste. Serve over pasta of your choice.

*Note:* Fennel is optional but it is more important if using ground beef. It is the unique seasoning in Italian sausage. For smoother consistency, place sauce in a food processor and blend until smooth.

NUTRITIONAL INFORMATION PER SERVING WITHOUT THE PASTA

Calories 200; Fat 9 gm.; Protein 11 gm.; Carbohydrate 17 gm.;
Cholesterol 30 mg.; Fiber 2.8 gm. (medium)

# MEATLESS
# MAIN COURSES
## (No Meat, Poultry, or Fish)

❖

*Angel Hair Pasta with Garlic and Olive Oil*

*Corn Pudding*

*Crustless Mexican Quiche*

*French Toast*

*Linguine Parmesan*

*Marinara Sauce*

*Mexican Macaroni Salad*

*Noodles Romanoff*

*Orange-Marinated Grilled Tofu*

*Pasta with Broccoli and Red Peppers in Peanut Sauce*

*Potato-Vegetable Bake*

*Puffy Omelet*

*Spinach Crock-Pot Casserole*

*Spinach, Feta Cheese, and Noodle Squares*

*Zucchini Casserole*

# Angel Hair Pasta with Garlic and Olive Oil

❖

*An easy, light pasta dish.*

❖ SERVES 4 ❖
Recipe texture: Easy to chew

8 ounces angel hair pasta or pasta of your choice
2 tablespoons olive oil, divided
3 cloves garlic, finely minced
2 cups fat-free chicken broth
½ teaspoon nutmeg
¼ cup finely chopped fresh basil or parsley

¼ teaspoon freshly ground pepper
1 tablespoon cornstarch
2 tablespoons water
salt to taste
½ cup freshly grated Parmesan cheese

Cook pasta in boiling water just until tender. Do not overcook. Drain pasta, then return it to the pan and toss with 1 tablespoon of olive oil. While pasta is cooking, heat 1 tablespoon oil in a small frying pan. Add garlic and cook over medium heat for 1 to 2 minutes. Do not brown the garlic. Add the chicken broth, nutmeg, basil, and pepper. Bring to a boil and simmer for 5 to 10 minutes.

Mix cornstarch with 2 tablespoons water and add to the pan. Bring to a boil, stirring constantly, until mixture thickens slightly. Add salt to taste. Add the chicken broth mixture to the pasta and toss quickly. Serve pasta in heated individual pasta bowls. Top with grated cheese.

*Note:* For a different taste, add 1 tablespoon fresh lemon juice to the chicken broth mixture.

NUTRITIONAL INFORMATION PER SERVING
Calories 315; Fat 10 gm.; Protein 12 gm.; Carbohydrate 44 gm.;
Cholesterol 10 mg.; Fiber 1.5 gm. (medium)

# Corn Pudding

❖

*This can also be served as a side dish. Kids love it, too.*

❖ SERVES 4 ❖

Recipe texture: Very easy to chew;
Soft and smooth if blended completely

¼  cup chopped onion
1   cup fat-free milk
2   eggs
1   tablespoon flour

½  teaspoon salt
¼  teaspoon white pepper
1   15-ounce can corn, drained

Preheat oven to 325 degrees. Butter an 8 × 8-inch baking pan. In a food processor or blender, combine onion, milk, eggs, flour, salt, and pepper. Blend until smooth. Add corn and blend briefly. Some corn may remain intact or if desired, continue to blend until smooth. Pour into baking pan. Bake for 30 to 40 minutes or until knife inserted in the center comes out clean.

*Note:* For a creamier texture, use 2% milk or whole milk.

NUTRITIONAL INFORMATION PER SERVING
Calories 185; Fat 3 gm.; Protein 8 gm.; Carbohydrate 32 gm.;
Cholesterol 90 mg.; Fiber 4 gm. (high)

# Crustless Mexican Quiche

❖

*This has lots of flavor but is not fiery hot.*

❖ SERVES 4 ❖

Recipe texture: Easy to chew;
Very easy to chew if egg mixture is blended smooth

5 large eggs
½ teaspoon baking powder
¼ cup flour
¼ teaspoon salt
¼ teaspoon pepper
1 cup low-fat small-curd cottage cheese

8 ounces low-fat shredded Monterey Jack and cheddar cheese blend
2 tablespoons butter or margarine, melted
1 4-ounce can green chiles, diced
1 cup salsa

Preheat oven to 350 degrees. Butter a 9-inch pie pan. In a large bowl, beat eggs until light and lemon-colored. Add baking powder, flour, salt, pepper, cottage cheese, shredded cheese, butter, and chilies. Beat until well mixed. (For a smoother consistency, blend egg mixture in a food processor.) Pour into pie pan. Bake for 40 to 50 minutes or until a knife inserted in the middle comes out clean. Allow to sit for 10 minutes before serving. Serve with salsa on the side.

*Note:* For less cholesterol and fat, use liquid egg substitute instead of eggs.

NUTRITIONAL INFORMATION PER SERVING
Calories 380; Fat 22 gm.; Protein 31 gm.; Carbohydrate 15 gm.;
Cholesterol 275 mg.; Fiber 1.1 gm. (medium)

# French Toast

❖

*Prepare this the night before for an easy breakfast or brunch.*

❖ SERVES 4 ❖

Recipe texture: Easy to chew;
Very easy to chew if made with crustless bread

| | | | |
|---|---|---|---|
| ½ | loaf French bread | ¼ | teaspoon salt |
| 4 | eggs | ¼ | teaspoon nutmeg |
| 1½ | cups fat-free milk | 1 | teaspoon vanilla |
| 1 | tablespoon sugar | 2 | tablespoons butter or margarine |

Heavily butter an 8 × 8-inch nonstick or glass baking pan. Cut French bread into 1-inch-thick slices. Arrange slices to fill pan in one layer. In a medium bowl, combine eggs, milk, sugar, salt, nutmeg, and vanilla. Beat well. Pour over bread. Dot with thin slices butter. Cover and refrigerate several hours or overnight. When ready to bake, preheat oven to 350 degrees. Bake, uncovered, for 30 to 45 minutes or until egg mixture is set and bread is lightly browned.

*Note:* Regular white bread can be substituted for the French bread. Cut off crusts if desired.

NUTRITIONAL INFORMATION PER SERVING
Calories 300; Fat 11 gm.; Protein 13 gm.; Carbohydrate 38 gm.;
Cholesterol 200 mg.; Fiber 1.6 gm. (medium)

# *Linguine Parmesan*

❖

*This is a great dish when you are in the mood
for something plain and simple.*

❖ SERVES 4 ❖

Recipe texture: Easy to chew

| | |
|---|---|
| 8 ounces linguine or other pasta | 1 cup shredded low-fat Monterey Jack and Colby cheese blend |
| 2 tablespoons butter or margarine | |
| 3 tablespoons flour | ½ cup grated Parmesan cheese, divided |
| ¼ teaspoon salt | |
| ⅛ teaspoon white pepper | 2 teaspoons lemon juice |
| 1½ cups fat-free milk | |

Cook linguine according to package directions until al dente. Drain and set aside. While pasta is cooking, melt butter in a medium saucepan. Add flour and stir over medium heat for 2 minutes. Add salt, pepper, and milk. Cook over medium heat, stirring constantly, until mixture comes to a boil. Continue to cook 1 to 2 minutes or until thickened. Remove from heat. Add shredded cheese, ¼ cup Parmesan cheese, and lemon juice. Stir until cheese is melted. Pour over warm linguine and toss until well mixed. Top with remaining Parmesan cheese.

*Note:* In place of the Monterey Jack and Colby cheese blend, use any cheese of your choice. Add additional milk for a thinner sauce.

NUTRITIONAL INFORMATION PER SERVING

Calories 445; Fat 15 gm.; Protein 24 gm.; Carbohydrate 53 gm.;
Cholesterol 45 mg.; Fiber 1.5 gm. (medium)

# Marinara Sauce

························· ❖ ·························

*Real homemade flavor, yet so easy. This is a great recipe to make ahead; it keeps for days in the refrigerator or it can be frozen. Just reheat and toss with pasta for a quick supper.*

❖ SERVES 4 ❖

Recipe texture: Very easy to chew;
Soft and smooth if blended

| | | | |
|---|---|---|---|
| 1 | tablespoon olive oil | 2 | bay leaves |
| 1 | large onion, finely chopped | 1 | teaspoon dried basil |
| 3 | cloves garlic, minced | ½ | teaspoon oregano |
| 2 | 15-ounce cans tomato sauce | ¼ | teaspoon thyme |
| 2 | 15-ounce cans Italian-style stewed tomatoes | ½ | teaspoon fresh ground pepper |
| ½ | cup water | 1 | teaspoon sugar |
| | | | salt to taste |

Heat oil in a large heavy saucepan. Add onion and cook over medium heat until translucent. Add garlic and cook 1 minute. Add tomato sauce, stewed tomatoes, water, bay leaves, basil, oregano, thyme, and pepper. Bring to a boil. Reduce heat and simmer slowly for about 1 hour or until sauce reaches desired thickness. Add sugar and salt to taste. Remove bay leaves. Add additional water if sauce is too thick. Serve over pasta.

*Note:* For a smoother sauce, place in a food processor or use an immersion blender and blend until desired consistency.

·················································

NUTRITIONAL INFORMATION PER SERVING WITHOUT PASTA

Calories 175; Fat 4 gm.; Protein 6 gm.; Carbohydrate 29 gm.;
Cholesterol 0 mg.; Fiber 5 gm. (very high)

# *Mexican Macaroni Salad*

❖

*Some like it hot!*

❖ SERVES 6 ❖

Recipe texture: Easy to chew

8  ounces elbow macaroni
(2½ cups)
1  15-ounce can hot chili beans,
drained and rinsed

½  red bell pepper, finely diced
6  ounces reduced-fat mozzarella
cheese, diced in ¼-inch pieces

**Dressing**
½  cup fat-free or low-fat
mayonnaise
¼  cup fat-free sour cream
¼  cup finely chopped onion
½  teaspoon chili powder

¼  teaspoon cumin
⅛  teaspoon garlic powder
dash hot pepper sauce
salt and freshly ground pepper to
taste

Cook macaroni in boiling salted water just until tender. Do not over-cook. Drain macaroni and rinse immediately under cold running water. Drain well. In a large bowl, combine macaroni, chili beans, bell pepper, and cheese. In a small bowl, combine mayonnaise, sour cream, onion, chili powder, cumin, garlic powder, hot pepper sauce, salt, and pepper. Combine with macaroni mixture. Gently mix well. Adjust seasoning with extra salt, pepper, and hot pepper sauce if desired. Refrigerate until ready to serve.

*Note:* For a milder dish, substitute canned kidney beans for the hot chili beans, omit the hot pepper sauce, and season to taste.

NUTRITIONAL INFORMATION PER SERVING
Calories 300; Fat 5 gm.; Protein 16 gm.; Carbohydrate 47 gm.;
Cholesterol 15 mg.; Fiber 6 gm. (very high)

# Noodles Romanoff

❖

*This easy entrée can also be served as a side dish
with grilled or roasted meats.*

❖ SERVES 4 ❖

Recipe texture: Easy to chew;
Very easy to chew with blended sauce

| | |
|---|---|
| 8   ounces noodles | ½   teaspoon Worcestershire sauce |
| 1   cup low-fat cottage cheese | dash Tabasco sauce |
| 1   cup fat-free sour cream | ½   cup grated Parmesan cheese, |
| ¼   cup diced onion |      divided |
| ¼   teaspoon garlic powder | ¼   cup milk (optional) |
| ½   teaspoon salt | paprika for garnish |

Cook noodles according to package directions until al dente. Drain
well and place back in the pan. In a medium bowl, combine cottage
cheese, sour cream, onion, garlic powder, salt, Worcestershire sauce,
Tabasco, and ¼ cup Parmesan cheese. Spoon into pan with noodles.
Place over medium heat and heat through. Add milk if thinner consistency is desired. Top individual servings with remaining Parmesan cheese and garnish with paprika.

*Note:* For a smoother sauce, blend cottage cheese, sour cream, and
onions together in a food processor.

NUTRITIONAL INFORMATION PER SERVING
Calories 355; Fat 6 gm.; Protein 24 gm.; Carbohydrate 52 gm.;
Cholesterol 70 mg.; Fiber 1.5 gm. (medium)

# *Orange-Marinated Grilled Tofu*

❖

*This marinade is also great for chicken and seafood.*

❖ SERVES 4 ❖

Recipe texture: Soft and smooth

24 ounces extra-firm low-fat tofu
1 cup orange juice
2 tablespoons lime juice (optional)
2 tablespoons sesame oil
3 tablespoons olive oil
¼ cup soy sauce

¼ cup dry sherry wine
2 cloves garlic, minced
1 teaspoon oregano
¼ teaspoon freshly ground pepper
dash salt

Cut tofu into bite-size pieces and place in a bowl or zip-top plastic bag. In a bowl or jar, combine all remaining ingredients. Pour marinade over the tofu, making sure the tofu is completely covered. Refrigerate for 15 to 30 minutes. Remove tofu from marinade and grill, broil, or sauté as desired.

NUTRITIONAL INFORMATION PER SERVING

Calories 100; Fat 2 gm.; Protein 16 gm.; Carbohydrate 7 gm.;
Cholesterol 0 mg.; Fiber 0.6 gm. (low)

# Pasta with Broccoli and Red Peppers in Peanut Sauce

❖

*This is a colorful dish with an unusual sauce
that has a subtle peanut flavor.*

❖ SERVES 4 ❖

Recipe texture: Easy to chew

**Sauce**

⅔ cup low-fat chicken broth
⅓ cup creamy peanut butter
3 tablespoons teriyaki sauce
1 tablespoon brown sugar

1 tablespoon lime juice
½ teaspoon garlic powder
⅛ teaspoon red pepper flakes, or
   more to taste

**Pasta and Vegetables**

½ cup chopped green onions
1 cup thinly sliced carrots
2 cups broccoli florets

1 medium red pepper, thinly sliced
6 cups cooked linguine or
   spaghetti

Combine all of the sauce ingredients in a small saucepan. Bring to a boil, stirring constantly. Remove from heat and set aside.

Place ½ cup of the sauce in a medium skillet. Add onions, carrots, broccoli, and red pepper. Cover and cook over medium heat until vegetables are crisp-tender. In a large serving bowl, combine vegetables and cooked warm pasta. Pour in desired amount of sauce and toss gently until well mixed.

*Added bonus:* 150 mcg. folate

NUTRITIONAL INFORMATION PER SERVING

Calories 530; Fat 16 gm.; Protein 20 gm.; Carbohydrate 77 gm.;
Cholesterol 0 mg.; Fiber 7 gm. (very high)

# *Potato-Vegetable Bake*

❖ ‧‧‧‧‧‧‧‧‧‧‧‧‧‧‧‧‧‧‧‧‧‧‧‧‧‧‧‧‧‧‧‧ ❖ ‧‧‧‧‧‧‧‧‧‧‧‧‧‧‧‧‧‧‧‧‧‧‧‧‧‧‧‧‧‧‧‧ ❖

*Choose the vegetables that work best for you
for this tasty casserole.*

❖ SERVES 8 ❖

Recipe texture: Easy to chew

| | |
|---|---|
| 1 tablespoon olive oil | 1 teaspoon dry mustard |
| 2 medium leeks, white and light green parts only, finely sliced | 1 tablespoon Italian seasoning |
| | ½ teaspoon cumin |
| 2 cups mixed vegetables, cut in small pieces | ¾ cup roasted red peppers, diced |
| 8 large eggs | 1 32-ounce package frozen southern-style hash brown potatoes |
| 1½ cups evaporated fat-free milk | |
| ½ cup fat-free milk | |
| 1½ teaspoons salt | 6 ounces shredded low-fat cheddar cheese, divided |
| 1 teaspoon pepper | |

Butter a 9 × 13-inch baking pan. Heat oil in a medium skillet. Add leeks and cook until tender. Add vegetables and 2 tablespoons water. Cover pan and cook just until vegetables are crisp-tender. Set aside.

In a large mixing bowl, combine eggs, evaporated milk, fat-free milk, salt, pepper, dry mustard, Italian seasoning, and cumin. Beat well. Stir in leeks and vegetables, roasted red peppers, potatoes, and ½ of the cheese. Pour into baking pan. Cover and refrigerate at least 8 hours or overnight.

*(continued)*

## *Potato-Vegetable Bake (continued)*

Preheat oven to 350 degrees. Bake, covered, for 45 minutes. Uncover and top with remaining 3 ounces of cheese. Bake an additional 20 to 30 minutes or until center is set. Let stand 10 minutes before serving. For extra zest, serve with tomato salsa.

*Note:* Southern-style hash brown potatoes are cut into small cubes. Country-style hash browns may also be used.

NUTRITIONAL INFORMATION PER SERVING

Calories 290; Fat 10 gm.; Protein 17 gm.; Carbohydrate 33 gm.; Cholesterol 200 mg.; Fiber 1.3 gm. (medium)

# *Puffy Omelet*

❖

*Serve this special fluffy omelet for breakfast or lunch.*

❖ SERVES 2 ❖

Recipe texture: Soft and smooth

| | |
|---|---|
| 4 large eggs, separated | ⅛ teaspoon pepper |
| ¼ cup water | 1 tablespoon butter or margarine |
| ¼ teaspoon salt | |

Preheat oven to 325 degrees. In a medium bowl, beat egg whites with water and salt until stiff but not dry. In another small bowl, beat egg yolks with pepper until thick and lemon-colored. Fold into egg whites. In a heavy 10-inch ovenproof skillet, melt butter until hot enough to sizzle a drop of water. Pour omelet mixture into skillet. Reduce heat. Cook slowly about 5 minutes or until puffy and lightly browned on bottom. (Lift omelet at edge with spatula to judge color.) Place in oven. Bake 10 to 15 minutes or until knife inserted in center comes out clean. To serve, tip skillet and loosen omelet by slipping spatula under and folding omelet in half without breaking.

NUTRITIONAL INFORMATION PER SERVING

Calories 170; Fat 14 gm.; Protein 10 gm.; Carbohydrate 1 gm.;
Cholesterol 380 mg.; Fiber 0 gm.

# Spinach Crock-Pot Casserole

❖

*A great meal for the spinach lover.*

❖ SERVES 8 ❖

Recipe texture: Very easy to chew;
Easy to chew if mushrooms are added

2  10-ounce packages frozen chopped spinach, thawed
2  cups low-fat small-curd cottage cheese
¼  cup butter or margarine, cut in small cubes

1½ cups shredded cheddar cheese
3  large eggs, lightly beaten
¼  cup flour
1  teaspoon salt
½  teaspoon pepper
dash hot pepper sauce

Grease well a slow-cooking Crock-Pot. Squeeze spinach dry and place in a large mixing bowl. Add all remaining ingredients and mix well. Pour into Crock-Pot. Cover and cook on high for 1 hour. Reduce heat to low and continue cooking for 4 to 5 hours.

*Note:* This is good with canned or sautéed mushrooms added.

NUTRITIONAL INFORMATION PER SERVING
Calories 235; Fat 15 gm.; Protein 17 gm.; Carbohydrate 8 gm.;
Cholesterol 110 mg.; Fiber 2.3 gm. (medium)

# *Spinach, Feta Cheese, and Noodle Squares*

❖

*This dish can be either a tasty meatless meal or a side dish. It can also be cut in small pieces and served as bite-size appetizers.*

❖ SERVES 8 ❖

Recipe texture: Easy to chew

| | |
|---|---|
| 1 tablespoon olive oil | 1 cup low-fat cottage cheese |
| 1 large onion, finely chopped | ½ cup freshly grated Parmesan |
| 4 cloves garlic, minced | cheese, divided |
| 1 10-ounce package frozen spinach, thawed and squeezed dry | ½ teaspoon fresh ground pepper |
| | ¼ teaspoon crushed red pepper |
| | ½ teaspoon oregano |
| 2 eggs, lightly beaten | 1 pound fine egg noodles |
| 8 ounces feta cheese, crumbled | butter-flavor cooking spray |

Preheat oven to 375 degrees. Butter a 9 × 13-inch nonstick baking pan. Heat oil in a medium skillet. Add onions and cook over medium heat until translucent. Add garlic and cook 1 minute. Remove from heat. In a medium bowl combine onions and garlic with spinach, eggs, feta cheese, cottage cheese, ¼ cup Parmesan cheese, pepper, crushed red pepper, and oregano. Stir until well mixed. Cook noodles in a large pot of salted water for 3 to 4 minutes or until al dente. (Do not overcook noodles.) Drain well. Spoon one-half of the noodles into the baking pan. Press down with back of the spoon. Spoon spinach mixture over the noodles and smooth out evenly. Arrange

*(continued)*

## *Spinach, Feta Cheese, and Noodle Squares (continued)*

remaining noodles on top. Press down with back of the spoon. Spray lightly with butter-flavor cooking spray. Sprinkle with remaining Parmesan cheese. Bake for 30 minutes or until golden brown. Cool 10 to 20 minutes before cutting.

*Note:* To serve four, prepare one-half of the recipe in an 8 × 8-inch pan.

........................................................................................

NUTRITIONAL INFORMATION PER SERVING
Calories 380; Fat 13 gm.; Protein 20 gm.; Carbohydrate 45 gm.;
Cholesterol 130 mg.; Fiber 3 gm. (high)

# *Zucchini Casserole*

❖

*This can be served as a meatless entrée
or as a vegetable side dish.*

❖ SERVES 8 ❖

Recipe texture: Easy to chew;
Very easy to chew if vegetables are blended

| | | | |
|---|---|---|---|
| 2 | tablespoons butter or margarine | 2½ | cups herb-seasoned stuffing cubes, divided |
| 6 | cups sliced fresh zucchini (about 8 medium) | 1 | 10¾-ounce can condensed cream of mushroom soup |
| 1 | cup shredded carrots | ½ | cup fat-free sour cream |
| ½ | cup finely chopped onion | | butter spray |
| ¼ | teaspoon salt | | |
| ¼ | teaspoon pepper | | |

Preheat oven to 350 degrees. Butter a 1½ quart casserole. Melt butter in a large skillet. Add zucchini, carrots, and onions. Cook until vegetables are crisp-tender. Remove from heat. Add salt, pepper, 1½ cups of the stuffing cubes, soup, and sour cream. Stir to mix well. Spoon into casserole. Top with remaining stuffing cubes. Spray with butter spray. Bake for 30 to 40 minutes or until heated through.

*Note:* For a smoother consistency, place sautéed vegetables in a food processor and blend until smooth.

NUTRITIONAL INFORMATION PER SERVING
Calories 190; Fat 5 gm.; Protein 7 gm.; Carbohydrate 35 gm.;
Cholesterol 10 mg.; Fiber 1.7 gm. (medium)

# SIDE DISHES

❖

Brown Sugar Baked Fruit

Deviled Eggs

Jell-O Jigglers

Lemon Bread

Noodle Pudding (Kugel)

Noodle Ring

Peachy Fruit Salad

Sautéed Apples

Spätzle

Speedy Tomato Aspic

# *Brown Sugar Baked Fruit*

•••••••••••••••••••••••••••••••••••• ❖ ••••••••••••••••••••••••••••••••••••

*A good way to dress up canned fruits.*

❖ SERVES 8 ❖

Recipe texture: Easy to chew;
Soft and smooth if blended

| | | |
|---|---|---|
| 1 | 15-ounce can sliced peaches, well drained | $\frac{1}{3}$ cup butter or margarine |
| 1 | 15-ounce can pear halves, well drained | $\frac{3}{4}$ cup brown sugar |
| 1 | 8-ounce can pineapple chunks, well drained | 1 teaspoon curry powder |

Preheat oven to 325 degrees. Arrange peaches, pears, and pineapple in a 1½-quart baking dish. In a small saucepan, combine butter, brown sugar, and curry powder. Melt over low heat. Pour over fruit. Bake for 30 to 45 minutes.

*Note:* For a smoother consistency, place fruit in a food processor and blend until smooth.

•••••••••••••••••••••••••••••••••••••••••••••••••••••••••••••••••••••••••

NUTRITIONAL INFORMATION PER SERVING
Calories 215; Fat 7 gm.; Protein 1 gm.; Carbohydrate 37 gm.;
Cholesterol 20 mg.; Fiber 2 gm. (medium)

# Deviled Eggs

......................................... ❖ ........................................

*An easy-to-enjoy old favorite.*

❖ SERVES 3 ❖

Recipe texture: Very easy to chew;
Soft and smooth for the egg yolk portion

3   hard-cooked eggs
3   tablespoons fat-free half-and-half
1   tablespoon sour cream
½   teaspoon mustard
¼   teaspoon pepper

¼   teaspoon salt
1   tablespoon minced chives
     (optional)
dash paprika

Peel hard-cooked eggs and cut in half. Scoop out yolks and mix with half-and-half, sour cream, mustard, pepper, and salt, and chives if desired. Mix well. Adjust seasoning to taste. Spoon yolk mixture back into egg whites. Sprinkle with paprika.

......................................................................................

NUTRITIONAL INFORMATION PER SERVING

Calories 125; Fat 11 gm.; Protein 6 gm.; Carbohydrate 1 gm.;
Cholesterol 200 mg.; Fiber 0 gm.

# *Jell-O Jigglers*

❖

*This treat will bring back childhood memories.*

❖ SERVES 12 ❖

Recipe texture: Soft and smooth

4   3-ounce packages Jell-O, any        2½ cups boiling water
flavor

In a large bowl, combine Jell-O powder with boiling water. Stir for 3 minutes or until gelatin is completely dissolved. Pour into a 9 × 13-inch pan. Refrigerate until set. Cut into small squares or shapes.

*Note:* Substitute fruit juice for part of the water, if desired.

NUTRITIONAL INFORMATION PER SERVING
Calories 110; Fat 0 gm.; Protein 2 gm.; Carbohydrate 26 gm.;
Cholesterol 0 mg.; Fiber 0 gm.

# Lemon Bread

❖

*This may be the easiest bread you will ever make. It is light
in texture with a marvelous lemon flavor. Yogurt takes the
place of oil in this recipe, making it low in fat. Serve it for
breakfast, for brunch, or with tea in the afternoon.*

❖ SERVES 20 ❖

Recipe texture: Very easy to chew

4   eggs
1   box (18 ounces) lemon cake mix
    with pudding in mix
1   3-ounce package instant lemon
    pudding mix

½   cup plain low-fat yogurt
1   cup hot water

Preheat oven to 325 degrees. Grease two 7½ × 3¾-inch loaf pans.

Beat eggs in a large mixing bowl. Stir in cake mix, pudding mix,
yogurt, and water. Mix well. Pour into loaf pans. Bake for 50 to 60
minutes if using large pans, or 40 to 50 minutes for small pans.
Bake until lightly brown and set in the middle.

*Note:* If desired, substitute ½ cup canola oil for the yogurt.

NUTRITIONAL INFORMATION PER SERVING

Calories 140; Fat 4 gm.; Protein 2 gm.; Carbohydrate 24 gm.;
Cholesterol 35 mg.; Fiber 0 gm.

# Noodle Pudding (Kugel)

····················· ❖ ·····················

*This is a traditional German side dish. With a slight sweetness, it complements chicken and pork dishes.*

❖ SERVES 8 ❖

Recipe texture: Easy to chew

6   ounces (3 cups) medium egg noodles
1   cup seedless white raisins (optional)
⅓   cup butter or margarine, melted
3   large eggs, beaten
⅓   cup sugar

¼   cup orange juice
1   cup low-fat sour cream
1   cup low-fat, small-curd cottage cheese
1   tablespoon vanilla
½   teaspoon allspice or nutmeg

Preheat oven to 350 degrees. Butter a deep 2-quart baking dish. Cook noodles in boiling salted water to al dente. Drain well and set aside. In a large bowl, combine all remaining ingredients. Beat until well mixed. Stir in noodles. Spoon into baking dish. Bake, uncovered, for 45 to 55 minutes or until set in the middle.

*Note:* There will be crispy noodles on the top of the baked dish but the inside portions will be soft.

··········································································

NUTRITIONAL INFORMATION PER SERVING

Calories 295; Fat 11 gm.; Protein 9 gm.; Carbohydrate 40 gm.; Cholesterol 115 mg.; Fiber 1.3 gm. (medium)

# Noodle Ring

❖

*An easy-to-enjoy noodle side dish.*

❖ SERVES 6 ❖

Recipe texture: Very easy to eat

| | |
|---|---|
| 8   ounces noodles | ½  teaspoon salt |
| ¾  cup fat-free milk | ¼  teaspoon white pepper |
| 3   eggs, lightly beaten | |
| 1   tablespoon butter or margarine, melted | |

Preheat oven to 350 degrees. Butter a 1½-quart ring mold or an 8 × 8-inch baking pan. Cook noodles in boiling salted water until al dente. Drain well. Spoon into pan. In a large bowl, combine milk, eggs, butter, salt, and pepper. Mix well. Pour over noodles in pan. Bake for 30 minutes or until set.

*Note:* For extra flavor, add herbs of your choice.

NUTRITIONAL INFORMATION PER SERVING

Calories 195; Fat 5 gm.; Protein 9 gm.; Carbohydrate 28 gm.; Cholesterol 135 mg.; Fiber 1 gm. (medium)

# *Peachy Fruit Salad*

......................................... ❖ .........................................

*This salad has a very attractive shiny appearance. Use any canned fruits you like.*

❖ SERVES 8 ❖

Recipe texture: Easy to chew

1   15-ounce can pineapple tidbits
1   15-ounce can peaches
1   15-ounce can pears

1   10-ounce can mandarin oranges
1   21-ounce can peach pie filling
1   large banana, sliced (optional)

Drain all canned fruits and combine in a large bowl. Stir in peach pie filling. Store in refrigerator. When ready to serve, stir in fresh bananas if desired.

.........................................................................................................

NUTRITIONAL INFORMATION PER SERVING

Calories 185; Fat 0 gm.; Protein 1 gm.; Carbohydrate 45 gm.;
Cholesterol 0 mg.; Fiber 3 gm. (high)

# Sautéed Apples

❖

*Cinnamon and apples just go together hand-in-hand. Serve as a side dish with pork or poultry. These apples are also delicious as a dessert, served over ice cream or frozen yogurt.*

❖ SERVES 8 ❖

Recipe texture: Easy to chew;
Soft and smooth if blended

3  tablespoons butter or margarine
6  cups peeled, sliced apples (about
   2 pounds)
½  cup brown sugar

½  teaspoon cinnamon
¼  teaspoon nutmeg
¼  cup apple juice (optional)

Melt butter in a large skillet. Add apples and cook over medium-high heat until tender. Stir in sugar, cinnamon, and nutmeg. Cook for 2 to 3 minutes until sugar melts. Add apple juice if a thinner sauce is desired.

*Note:* Use an all-purpose apple, such as Macintosh or Yellow Delicious. For a smoother consistency, place sautéed apples in a food processor, and process until smooth.

NUTRITIONAL INFORMATION PER SERVING

Calories 140; Fat 4 gm.; Protein 0 gm.; Carbohydrate 26 gm.;
Cholesterol 10 mg.; Fiber 1.9 gm. (medium)

# *Spätzle*

❖

*Surprise yourself and your family
with a homemade dish from the past.*

❖ SERVES 6 ❖

Recipe texture: Very easy to chew

| | |
|---|---|
| 2  cups flour | ¼  cup minced fresh parsley, divided |
| 3  eggs | ¾  cup milk |
| 1  teaspoon salt | 2  tablespoons butter |
| ½  teaspoon white pepper | ½  cup seasoned bread crumbs |
| ¼  teaspoon nutmeg | (optional) |

Bring a pan of water to a boil. In a medium bowl, mix flour, eggs, salt, pepper, nutmeg, 1 tablespoon minced parsley, and enough milk to make a heavy dough. Drop very small pieces of dough into the boiling water. Cook for about 5 minutes or until dough is completely cooked. Stir occasionally. Remove spätzle with a slotted spoon and place in a colander. Rinse with cold water, drain well, and set aside. Melt butter in a nonstick skillet. Add the cooked spätzle and sauté over medium heat until golden brown. Add bread crumbs if desired and brown lightly. Sprinkle with remaining parsley. Serve as a side dish with meat or other German dishes.

NUTRITIONAL INFORMATION PER SERVING
Calories 260; Fat 6 gm.; Protein 10 gm.; Carbohydrate 43 gm.;
Cholesterol 100 mg.; Fiber 0.3 gm. (low)

# Speedy Tomato Aspic

❖

*Adds color and interest to any meal.*

❖ SERVES 4 ❖

Recipe texture: Soft and smooth

1½ cups V-8 vegetable juice          ½   cup cold water
1     3-ounce package lemon Jell-O

Heat vegetable juice until almost boiling. Add Jell-O and stir until dissolved. Remove from heat and add the cold water. Pour into gelatin mold. Chill until set.

NUTRITIONAL INFORMATION PER SERVING

Calories 100; Fat 0 gm.; Protein 2 gm.; Carbohydrate 23 gm.;
Cholesterol 0 mg.; Fiber 0.7 gm. (low)

# VEGETABLES

❖

*Beets in Lemon-Butter Pineapple Sauce*

*Bourbon Sweet Potatoes*

*Butternut Squash and Apple Bake*

*Honey-Ginger Carrots*

*Mashed Potatoes with Carrots*

*Parmesan Potatoes*

*Red Cabbage and Apples*

*Spicy Orange Beets*

*Spinach Soufflé*

*Sweet Potato Casserole*

# Beets in Lemon-Butter Pineapple Sauce

❖

*This is a great way to dress up beets.*

❖ SERVES 6 ❖

Recipe texture: Easy to chew

| | |
|---|---|
| 1   15-ounce can pineapple chunks in light syrup | 2   tablespoons butter or margarine |
| 2   tablespoons cornstarch | 2   tablespoons lemon juice |
| 1   30-ounces can beets, drained | salt and pepper to taste |

Drain pineapple and reserve the juice. Set pineapple chunks aside. Place juice in a measuring cup. Add enough water to the juice to make 1 cup of liquid. Add cornstarch and stir until smooth. Pour into medium saucepan. Cook, stirring constantly, over medium heat until mixture bubbles and thickens. Remove from the stove. Add beets, butter, lemon juice, and pineapple chunks. Return to stove to heat through. Add salt and pepper to taste.

NUTRITIONAL INFORMATION PER SERVING

Calories 125; Fat 4 gm.; Protein 1 gm.; Carbohydrate 22 gm.;
Cholesterol 10 mg.; Fiber 2 gm. (medium)

# *Bourbon Sweet Potatoes*

❖

*An old-fashioned recipe for a super-healthy vegetable.*

❖ SERVES 8 ❖

Recipe texture: Soft and smooth

2 pounds canned sweet potatoes, drained
2 tablespoons butter or margarine
¼ cup bourbon

⅓ cup orange juice
¼ cup brown sugar
½ teaspoon salt
½ teaspoon apple pie spice

Preheat oven to 350 degrees. Butter a 1½-quart casserole. Place sweet potatoes in large bowl. Add butter, bourbon, orange juice, brown sugar, salt, and apple pie spice. Using an electric beater, mix until fluffy and smooth. Spoon into baking dish. Bake 20 to 30 minutes or until heated through.

*Note:* Fresh sweet potatoes or yams can be used. Peel and cook in boiling water until tender.

NUTRITIONAL INFORMATION PER SERVING

Calories 170; Fat 4 gm.; Protein 2 gm.; Carbohydrate 31 gm.;
Cholesterol 10 mg.; Fiber 2.6 gm. (medium)

# Butternut Squash and Apple Bake

❖

*This is so good you could almost serve it for dessert.*

❖ SERVES 8 ❖

Recipe texture: Easy to chew;
Very easy to chew if apples are cut into small pieces;
Soft and smooth for the mashed squash portion

| | |
|---|---|
| 1   medium butternut squash (1½ pounds) | 1   tablespoon brown sugar |
| 1   tablespoon butter or margarine | 2   medium apples, peeled and cored |
| ½   teaspoon salt | ¼   teaspoon cinnamon |
| ¼   teaspoon pepper | 2   tablespoons sugar |

**Topping**

| | |
|---|---|
| 1   cup corn flakes, slightly crushed | 1   tablespoon butter, melted |
| ¼   cup chopped pecans, optional | 1   tablespoon brown sugar |

Peel squash and cut in half lengthwise; remove seeds. Cut into large pieces. Place in a large pan with 2 inches of water. Cover and boil gently over medium heat for 20 to 30 minutes or until squash is tender. Drain well. Add the butter, salt, pepper, and brown sugar. Mash with electric mixer. Set aside.

Preheat oven to 350 degrees. Butter a deep 9-inch round pie pan. Thinly slice apples and arrange in pan. Sprinkle with cinnamon and sugar. Spread mashed squash over apples. Combine topping ingredients in a small bowl. Sprinkle over squash. Bake for 25 to 30 minutes or until apples are tender.

NUTRITIONAL INFORMATION PER SERVING

Calories 125; Fat 4 gm.; Protein 1 gm.; Carbohydrate 22 gm.; Cholesterol 10 mg.; Fiber 1.2 gm. (medium)

# Honey-Ginger Carrots

❖

*Add a little sugar and spice to your carrots.*

❖ Serves 4 ❖

Recipe texture: Easy to chew;
Soft and smooth if blended

| | |
|---|---|
| 1 pound carrots, peeled and sliced | ¼ teaspoon ground ginger |
| ¼ cup honey | ½ teaspoon salt |
| 2 tablespoons sugar | 1 teaspoon grated lemon peel |
| 2 tablespoons butter or margarine | |

In a medium saucepan, cook carrots in boiling water for 10 minutes. Drain well. Add honey, sugar, butter, ginger, and salt. Cook, uncovered, over low heat, stirring occasionally, until carrots are tender and richly glazed (10 to 15 minutes). Stir in lemon peel. If desired, blend in a food processor.

NUTRITIONAL INFORMATION PER SERVING

Calories 180; Fat 5 gm.; Protein 1 gm.; Carbohydrate 33 gm.;
Cholesterol 15 mg.; Fiber 3.1 gm. (high)

# *Mashed Potatoes with Carrots*

❖

*The carrots add extra nutrients and help prevent
the potatoes from getting gummy.*

❖ SERVES 6 ❖

Recipe texture: Soft and smooth

5 medium potatoes, peeled and chopped
3 large carrots, peeled and chopped

½ cup milk
⅛ teaspoon white pepper
salt to taste

In a large saucepan, cook potatoes and carrots in boiling water until tender. Drain well. Add milk to pan. Using an electric mixer, whip potatoes and carrots until light and fluffy. Add extra milk if needed to make the desired consistency. Add pepper and salt to taste.

*Note:* Add butter or margarine if desired. Choose potatoes such as russet potatoes that do not get gummy and sticky when whipped.

NUTRITIONAL INFORMATION PER SERVING

Calories 200; Fat 0 gm.; Protein 5 gm.; Carbohydrate 45 gm.;
Cholesterol 0 mg.; Fiber 4.5 gm. (very high)

# *Parmesan Potatoes*

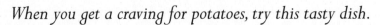

*When you get a craving for potatoes, try this tasty dish.*

❖ SERVES 6 ❖

Recipe texture: Easy to chew

¼ cup butter or margarine
1 medium onion, finely chopped
½ teaspoon salt
¼ teaspoon white pepper
⅛ teaspoon garlic powder
1 cup fat-free half-and-half

1 12-ounce package loose-packed frozen shredded hash browns, thawed
1 cup grated Parmesan cheese, divided
dash paprika

Preheat oven to 350 degrees. Butter a 7 × 11-inch baking pan. Melt butter in a medium skillet. Add onion and cook over medium heat until translucent. Add salt, pepper, garlic powder, and half-and-half. Heat through. Stir in hash brown potatoes. Add half of the cheese. Stir to mix. Spoon potatoes into prepared pan. Cover with foil and bake for 30 minutes. Remove foil and top with remaining cheese. Sprinkle with paprika. Return to oven and turn on the broiler. Broil until cheese melts and forms a crust.

NUTRITIONAL INFORMATION PER SERVING
Calories 300; Fat 19 gm.; Protein 10 gm.; Carbohydrate 21 gm.;
Cholesterol 40 mg.; Fiber 0.7 gm. (low)

# Red Cabbage and Apples

❖

*The lemon juice in this dish helps red cabbage keep its bright red color. This is an unusual combination of flavors that goes well with pork dishes.*

❖ SERVES 4 ❖

Recipe texture: Easy to chew

| | |
|---|---|
| 4 cups shredded red cabbage (about 1½ pounds) | ¼ cup red currant jelly |
| 2 teaspoons lemon juice | ¼ cup water |
| 2 medium apples, peeled and diced | 1 teaspoon salt |

Combine all ingredients in a large saucepan. Bring to a boil, then lower heat to medium and cook, partially covered, for 30 minutes, or until tender. Stir occasionally.

NUTRITIONAL INFORMATION PER SERVING

Calories 120; Fat 0 gm.; Protein 2 gm.; Carbohydrate 28 gm.;
Cholesterol 0 mg.; Fiber 4.2 gm. (high)

# Spicy Orange Beets

❖

*The flavors of orange and cloves complement the beets.*

❖ SERVES 6 ❖

Recipe texture: Very easy to chew;
Soft and smooth if blended

| | |
|---|---|
| 1 30-ounce can shredded beets, drained | ¼ cup orange juice |
| 1 tablespoon sugar | 2 tablespoons butter or margarine |
| ⅛ teaspoon ground cloves | 2 tablespoons grated orange peel (optional) |

In a large saucepan, combine beets, sugar, cloves, orange juice, and butter. Place over low heat until heated through. Garnish with orange peel. If desired, blend in a food processor.

NUTRITIONAL INFORMATION PER SERVING

Calories 90; Fat 4 gm.; Protein 1 gm.; Carbohydrate 12 gm.;
Cholesterol 0 mg.; Fiber 1.6 gm. (medium)

# *Spinach Soufflé*

❖

*This nutritious side dish
can also be served as a main course.*

❖ SERVES 6 ❖

Recipe texture: Easy to chew

2   10-ounce packages frozen
    chopped spinach, thawed and
    squeezed dry
2   cups low-fat cottage cheese or
    ricotta cheese
½   teaspoon salt

¼   teaspoon white pepper
⅛   teaspoon nutmeg
2   eggs, lightly beaten
1½  cups shredded low-fat cheddar
    cheese, divided

Preheat oven to 350 degrees. Butter a 7 × 11-inch baking pan. In a
large bowl, combine spinach, cottage cheese, salt, pepper, nutmeg,
eggs, and ½ cup cheddar cheese. Stir to mix well. Spoon into pan.
Bake for 40 to 50 minutes or until set. Remove from the oven. Top
with remaining cheese. Return to oven for 3 to 5 minutes or until the
cheese is melted. Let stand 5 to 10 minutes before serving.

NUTRITIONAL INFORMATION PER SERVING

Calories 175; Fat 7 gm.; Protein 21 gm.; Carbohydrate 7 gm.;
Cholesterol 85 mg.; Fiber 2.8 gm. (medium)

# Sweet Potato Casserole

❖

*What a sweet way to get your vitamin A.*

❖ SERVES 4 ❖

Recipe texture: Easy to chew

2   cups canned sweet potatoes,
    drained
¼   cup brown sugar
¼   cup fat-free milk
1   tablespoon butter or margarine,
    melted

1   teaspoon vanilla
½   teaspoon salt
1   egg, lightly beaten

**Topping**

¼   cup brown sugar
¼   cup flour

2   tablespoons butter or margarine,
    melted

Preheat oven to 350 degrees. Butter a 1½-quart casserole dish. In a medium bowl, combine sweet potatoes, brown sugar, milk, butter, vanilla, salt, and eggs. Beat with an electric mixer. Spoon into casserole dish.

For the topping, combine brown sugar, flour, and butter in a small bowl. Sprinkle over sweet potatoes. Bake for 20 to 30 minutes or until heated through.

NUTRITIONAL INFORMATION PER SERVING

Calories 270; Fat 9 gm.; Protein 3 gm.; Carbohydrate 45 gm.;
Cholesterol 70 mg.; Fiber 1.6 gm. (medium)

# SAUCES AND SPREADS

❖

Black Cherry Sauce

Blueberry Sauce

Cheese Sauce (Low-Fat)

Cranberry, Chili, and Cilantro Sauce

Curry Sauce

Guacamole

Hummus Spread

Mushroom Sauce

Parmesan Sauce

Smoked Salmon Pâté

Snappy Cocktail Sauce

Sweet-and-Sour Peach Sauce

Tarragon-Mustard Sauce

Warm Lemon Sauce

Yogamole

*Note:* The recipes in this section were chosen to give you ideas for adding moisture and flavor to your foods. Some of the sauces and spreads will complement dessert dishes; others will complement main course dishes.

# *Black Cherry Sauce*

❖

*Serve with chicken, duck, or Cornish hens.*

❖ SERVES 4 ❖

Recipe texture: Easy to chew if some of the cherries are left whole;
Soft and smooth if completely blended

1½ cups pitted sweet Bing cherries    pinch white pepper (optional)
    in juice
1    tablespoon port wine

Drain cherries and reserve the juice. Place cherries and ¼ cup of the
juice in a food processor or blender. Process until smooth. Pour into
small heavy saucepan. Add wine and bring to a boil. Cook over
medium heat about 10 minutes or until slightly thickened. Add pinch
of pepper if desired. Makes 1 cup.

*Note:* If desired, purée only ½ of the cherries and leave the others
whole.

NUTRITIONAL INFORMATION PER SERVING
Calories 50; Fat 0 gm.; Protein 1 gm.; Carbohydrate 13 gm.;
Cholesterol 0 mg.; Fiber 0.6 gm. (low)

# *Blueberry Sauce*

❖

*Serve over yogurt, ice cream, cheesecake, or fruits.*

❖ SERVES 4 ❖
Recipe texture: Soft and smooth

| | |
|---|---|
| 1 pint fresh blueberries | ¼ teaspoon allspice |
| ¼ cup apricot nectar | sugar to taste |
| 1 teaspoon lemon juice | |

In a blender or food processor, combine blueberries, apricot nectar, lemon juice, and allspice. Process until smooth. Add sugar to taste. Strain if desired. Makes 1½ cups.

NUTRITIONAL INFORMATION PER SERVING
Calories 50; Fat 0 gm.; Protein 1 gm.; Carbohydrate 12 gm.;
Cholesterol 0 mg.; Fiber 2 gm. (medium)

# Cheese Sauce (Low-Fat)

❖

*This makes cooked vegetables taste so good.*

❖ SERVES 8 ❖

Recipe texture: Soft and smooth

2 tablespoons butter or margarine
3 tablespoons flour
2 cups fat-free milk
4 ounces fat-free processed
  American cheese

¼ teaspoon white pepper
salt to taste

Melt butter in a small heavy saucepan. Add flour and cook over medium heat, stirring constantly with a wooden spoon for 2 minutes. Add milk and bring to a boil. Reduce heat and cook 2 minutes. Add cheese, pepper, and salt. Heat until cheese is melted, stirring constantly. Remove from heat until ready to serve. Rewarm before serving and add extra milk if sauce is too thick. Makes 2 cups.

NUTRITIONAL INFORMATION PER SERVING
Calories 75; Fat 3 gm.; Protein 7 gm.; Carbohydrate 5 gm.;
Cholesterol 10 mg.; Fiber 0 gm.

# Cranberry, Chili, and Cilantro Salsa

❖

*This will brighten up the flavor of poultry, pork, or fish.*

❖ SERVES 6 ❖

Recipe texture: Soft and smooth

| | | | |
|---|---|---|---|
| 1 | 12-ounce package fresh or frozen cranberries | 1 | small jalapeno pepper, seeded and minced |
| 1½ | cups water | ¼ | cup finely chopped sweet onions |
| 1 | cup sugar | ¼ | cup lime juice |
| 1 | clove garlic, minced | | dash salt |
| ¼ | cup fresh cilantro, minced | | dash pepper |

In a large saucepan, combine cranberries, water, and sugar. Bring to a boil, reduce heat, and partially cover. Simmer for 3 to 5 minutes or until cranberries begin to pop and are tender. Add remaining ingredients and cool to room temperature. Spoon into a food processor and process until smooth. Add additional sugar if desired. Makes 3 cups.

NUTRITIONAL INFORMATION PER SERVING

Calories 160; Fat 0 gm.; Protein 0.5 gm.; Carbohydrate 40 gm.;
Cholesterol 0 mg.; Fiber 2.6 gm. (medium)

# *Curry Sauce*

❖

*Use this sauce to add zest to cooked vegetables.*

❖ SERVES 4 ❖

Recipe texture: Soft and smooth

1 cup low-fat mayonnaise
1 tablespoon tarragon vinegar
1 tablespoon lemon juice
½ teaspoon Worcestershire sauce
1 teaspoon curry powder

dash thyme
1 tablespoon chili sauce (optional)
salt and freshly ground pepper to
  taste

Combine all ingredients in a small bowl. Cover and refrigerate until ready to serve. May be served chilled or at room temperature. Makes 1 cup.

NUTRITIONAL INFORMATION PER SERVING

Calories 100; Fat 4 gm.; Protein 0 gm.; Carbohydrate 16 gm.;
Cholesterol 0 mg.; Fiber 0 gm.

# *Guacamole*

❖

*Avocados are rich in the healthy monounsaturated fats.*

❖ SERVES 4 ❖

Recipe texture: Easy to chew;
Soft and smooth if completely blended

| | | | |
|---|---|---|---|
| 1 | small onion, chopped | 2 | medium avocados, peeled and chopped |
| 1 | clove garlic | | |
| 1 | tablespoon lime juice | 1 | medium tomato, seeded and chopped |
| ½ | cup fat-free sour cream | | |
| ¼ | teaspoon Worcestershire sauce | | Tabasco sauce to taste |
| ½ | teaspoon chili powder | | salt and pepper to taste |

In a food processor, combine onion, garlic, lime juice, sour cream, Worcestershire sauce, and chili powder. Process until smooth. Add avocado and tomatoes. Process briefly until desired consistency. Add Tabasco sauce, salt, and pepper to taste. Makes 1½ cups.

*Note:* If a thinner consistency is desired, add cream or milk.

NUTRITIONAL INFORMATION PER SERVING
Calories 170; Fat 11 gm.; Protein 4 gm.; Carbohydrate 14 gm.;
Cholesterol 3 mg.; Fiber 2.5 gm. (medium)

# Hummus Spread

❖

*This Middle Eastern staple is*
*traditionally served with pita bread.*

❖ SERVES 4 ❖
Recipe texture: Soft and smooth

1   15-ounce can garbanzo beans,
    drained
½  cup low-fat cottage cheese
2   tablespoons tahini (sesame-seed
    paste)
1   tablespoon lemon juice

½  teaspoon grated lemon peel
1   clove garlic
¼  teaspoon coriander (optional)
salt and freshly ground pepper to
    taste

Place all ingredients except salt and pepper in a food processor and
process until smooth. Add salt and pepper to taste. Store in the
refrigerator. Makes 1½ cups.

*Note:* For extra flavor and extra calories, add additional tahini. If a
thinner consistency is desired, stir in plain yogurt.

NUTRITIONAL INFORMATION PER SERVING
Calories 195; Fat 5 gm.; Protein 10 gm.; Carbohydrate 27 gm.;
Cholesterol 0 mg.; Fiber 5.2 gm. (very high)

# *Mushroom Sauce*

❖

*Mushrooms have a special flavoring component, glutamine,
that makes meat and vegetable dishes taste better.*

❖ SERVES 4 ❖

Recipe texture: Very easy to chew;
Soft and smooth if blended

| | | | |
|---|---|---|---|
| 1½ | cups finely chopped mushrooms | 1 | cup fat-free beef broth |
| 1 | tablespoon flour | 2 | teaspoons Worcestershire sauce |
| ½ | cup port wine | 1 | teaspoon tomato paste |
| ¼ | cup minced shallots | ⅛ | teaspoon rosemary |
| 1 | tablespoon balsamic vinegar | 1 | teaspoon Dijon mustard |

Combine mushrooms and flour in a plastic bag. Toss to mix well. Set
aside. Place wine and shallots in a small saucepan. Boil for about 3
minutes or until reduced by half. Add vinegar, broth, Worcestershire
sauce, tomato paste, and rosemary. Cook 1 minute. Add mushrooms
and cook for 3 minutes, stirring constantly. Stir in mustard.

Serve with beef or pork. Makes 1½ cups.

*Note:* For a smoother consistency, place in a food processor and
blend until smooth. If desired, the sauce may also be thickened with
a cornstarch and water mixture.

NUTRITIONAL INFORMATION PER SERVING
Calories 80; Fat 1 gm.; Protein 1 gm.; Carbohydrate 9 gm.;
Cholesterol 0 mg.; Fiber 0.4 gm. (low); Alcohol 5 gm.

# *Parmesan Sauce*

❖

*This sauce is good served over cooked vegetables or fish.*

❖ SERVES 6 ❖

Recipe texture: Soft and smooth

⅓  cup flour
3   cups fat-free milk, divided
¼  teaspoon nutmeg

1   cup grated Parmesan cheese
1   teaspoon butter or margarine
salt and freshly ground pepper

In a cup-sized shaker, combine flour and ¾ cup of milk. Shake until smooth. (If you don't have a shaker, combine flour with a small amount of milk. Whisk until smooth. Gradually add the remaining ¾ cup milk, whisking after each addition.) Pour flour and milk mixture into a small heavy saucepan. Add remaining 2¼ cups milk and nutmeg. Cook over medium heat, stirring constantly, until mixture comes to a boil. Cook for 1 more minute. Remove from heat and stir in cheese and butter. Stir until melted. Add salt and pepper to taste. Makes 3 cups.

NUTRITIONAL INFORMATION PER SERVING
Calories 150; Fat 6 gm.; Protein 12 gm.; Carbohydrate 12 gm.;
Cholesterol 15 mg.; Fiber 0 gm.

# Smoked Salmon Pâté

❖

*Serve this on bread or use it as a dip for cooked vegetables.*

❖ SERVES 8 ❖

Recipe texture: Soft and smooth

8 ounces low-fat cream cheese
¼ cup fat-free sour cream
2 tablespoons fresh parsley leaves

1 tablespoon Dijon mustard
4 ounces smoked salmon
salt and pepper to taste

In a food processor, combine cream cheese, sour cream, parsley, and mustard. Blend until smooth. Add salmon and process to desired consistency. Add salt and pepper to taste. Spoon into bowl, cover, and refrigerate. Makes 2 cups.

*Note:* If mixture is too thick, thin with extra sour cream or milk.

NUTRITIONAL INFORMATION PER SERVING
Calories 70; Fat 5 gm.; Protein 5 gm.; Carbohydrate 1 gm.;
Cholesterol 20 mg.; Fiber 0 gm.

# Snappy Cocktail Sauce

❖

*Perk up fish and shellfish with this zesty sauce.*

❖ SERVES 4 ❖

Recipe texture: Soft and smooth

| | |
|---|---|
| 1   cup ketchup | dash Tabasco sauce |
| 1   tablespoon horseradish | 1   teaspoon lemon juice |

Mix all ingredients together in a small bowl. Cover and refrigerate. It will keep for at least a week. Makes 1 cup.

*Note:* Some horseradish is extremely hot. Start out with a small amount and add more to taste for extra flavor.

NUTRITIONAL INFORMATION PER SERVING

Calories 90; Fat 2 gm.; Protein 1 gm.; Carbohydrate 17 gm.;
Cholesterol 5 mg.; Fiber 0.8 gm. (low)

# Sweet-and-Sour Peach Sauce

❖

*This unusual blend of interesting flavors*
*adds moistness and zest to chicken or pork.*

❖ SERVES 4 ❖

Recipe texture: Soft and smooth

½  tablespoon olive oil
½  cup chopped red onion
2   medium fresh peaches, pitted, peeled, and sliced
1   medium fresh tomato, peeled and chopped

½  teaspoon ground ginger
¼  cup orange juice
¼  cup cider vinegar
2½ tablespoons brown sugar
½  teaspoon allspice
salt and pepper to taste

Heat oil in a large nonstick skillet. Add onions and cook over medium heat until translucent. Add all remaining ingredients. Bring to a boil, reduce heat, and simmer for 20 to 30 minutes or until peaches are very tender. Place in a food processor and process until smooth. Makes 1½ cups.

NUTRITIONAL INFORMATION PER SERVING

Calories 90; Fat 2 gm.; Protein 1 gm.; Carbohydrate 17gm.;
Cholesterol 0 mg.; Fiber 1.3 gm. (medium)

# *Tarragon-Mustard Sauce*

❖

*Add a boost of flavor and moisture to chicken or fish dishes.*

❖ SERVES 2 ❖

Recipe texture: Soft and smooth

| | |
|---|---|
| 2 tablespoons flour | 2 teaspoons tarragon vinegar |
| 1 cup fat-free milk | salt and freshly ground pepper to |
| ⅛ teaspoon white pepper |    taste |
| 2 teaspoons dry mustard | 1 sprig fresh tarragon (optional) |

In a shaker or a small jar, mix flour and milk until smooth. Pour into small heavy saucepan. Bring to a boil over medium heat, stirring constantly. Boil gently for 2 minutes. Add white pepper, dry mustard, and vinegar. Add salt and pepper to taste. Store leftover sauce in a covered jar with a sprig of tarragon. Makes 1 cup.

NUTRITIONAL INFORMATION PER SERVING

Calories 75; Fat 1 gm.; Protein 5 gm.; Carbohydrate 12 gm.;
Cholesterol 2 mg.; Fiber 0 gm.

# *Warm Lemon Sauce*

*Serve this over cake, frozen yogurt, or ice cream.*

❖ SERVES 8 ❖

Recipe texture: Soft and smooth

| | |
|---|---|
| 1   cup sugar | ½   cup lemon juice |
| 1   tablespoon grated lemon peel | ½   cup water |
| 1½ tablespoons cornstarch | 2   teaspoons butter or margarine |

In a small saucepan, combine sugar, lemon peel, and cornstarch. Gradually whisk in lemon juice and water. Bring to a boil, stirring constantly until mixture is slightly thickened. Remove from heat and whisk in butter. Serve warm. Makes 1 cup.

NUTRITIONAL INFORMATION PER SERVING

Calories 120; Fat 1 gm.; Protein 0 gm.; Carbohydrate 28 gm.;
Cholesterol 3 mg.; Fiber 0 gm.

# *Yogamole*

❖

*Nutritious yogurt and avocado dip for cooked vegetables.*

❖ SERVES 4 ❖

Recipe texture: Very easy to chew;
Soft and smooth if completely blended

½ cup fat-free plain yogurt
1 large avocado, peeled and chopped
¼ cup diced onion
1 tablespoon lemon juice

¼ teaspoon cumin
dash Tabasco sauce
1 medium fresh tomato, seeded and finely chopped
dash salt and freshly ground pepper

In a food processor, combine yogurt, avocado, onion, lemon juice, cumin, and Tabasco. Process until smooth. Stir in tomato or, if desired, add tomato and process until smooth. Add salt and pepper to taste. Makes 1½ cups.

NUTRITIONAL INFORMATION PER SERVING
Calories 75; Fat 5 gm.; Protein 2 gm.; Carbohydrate 6 gm.;
Cholesterol 0 mg.; Fiber 1.3 gm. (medium)

# DESSERTS

❖

Apple Cake with Hot Buttered Rum Sauce

Apple Scotch Crisp

Bananas Foster

Bread Pudding

Buttermilk Pie

Caramel Cheesecake

Caramel Flan

Cheesecake Pie

Chess Pie

Chocolate Silk Pie

Classic Custard

Cocoa Fudge Dessert

Country Apple Coffee Cake

Crème Caramel

Custard Pie

Fudge Bottom Pie

Key Lime Pie

## DESSERTS *(continued)*

*Lemonade Cake*

*Lemon-Lime Supreme Refrigerator Cake*

*Lemon Pudding Cake*

*Mandarin Orange–Pineapple Cake*

*Mini Cheese Cakes*

*Peach Surprise*

*Pistachio Pudding Pie*

*Poached Pears with Chocolate Cranberry Sauce*

*Pumpkin Bars*

*Pumpkin Pie*

*Rhubarb Bread Pudding*

*Rhubarb Crumble*

*Rice Pudding*

*So Smooth Carrot Cake*

*Strawberry Delight*

# *Apple Cake with Hot Buttered Rum Sauce*

❖

*If you like something soft, moist, sweet, and warm you will love this dessert.*

❖ SERVES 10 ❖

Recipe texture: Easy to chew

| | |
|---|---|
| ¼  cup butter or margarine | ¼  teaspoon ground ginger |
| 1   cup sugar | ¼  teaspoon nutmeg |
| 1   egg | 1   teaspoon vanilla |
| ½  teaspoon salt | 1   cup flour |
| 1   teaspoon baking soda | 2   cups finely diced peeled apples |
| ½  teaspoon cinnamon | |

**Topping**

| | |
|---|---|
| ¼  cup fat-free evaporated milk | ½  cup brown sugar |
| 2   tablespoons butter or margarine | 1   tablespoon rum |

Preheat oven to 325 degrees. Butter a 7 × 11-inch baking pan. In a large bowl beat butter and sugar until creamy. Add egg and beat until smooth. Add salt, baking soda, cinnamon, ginger, nutmeg, and vanilla. Beat until well mixed. Stir in flour and mix just until smooth. Stir in apples. Pour into pan. Bake for 25 to 30 minutes or until cake is done. The cake should be lightly browned and the middle of cake should spring back when touched lightly with your finger.

For the topping, combine evaporated milk, butter, and brown sugar in a small saucepan. Stir over medium heat until mixture just

*(continued)*

## Apple Cake with Hot Buttered Rum Sauce
### *(continued)*

comes to a boil. Immediately remove from heat. (Mixture will curdle if allowed to boil rapidly.) Stir in rum. Serve warm over individual pieces of cake.

*Note:* To use a 9 × 13-inch pan, prepare 1½ times the recipe. Will serve 15.

NUTRITIONAL INFORMATION PER SERVING
Calories 250; Fat 9 gm.; Protein 2 gm.; Carbohydrate 40 gm.;
Cholesterol 35 mg.; Fiber 1.1 gm. (medium)

# Apple Scotch Crisp

❖

*Tastes like a caramel apple but it is softer.*

❖ Serves 8 ❖

Recipe texture: Easy to chew

| | |
|---|---|
| 1   3.5-ounce package butterscotch pudding mix | ¼ cup fat-free milk |
| ½ cup brown sugar | ½ cup water |
| 1   tablespoon flour | 6   cups peeled, sliced apples (about 6 medium) |

**Topping**

| | |
|---|---|
| ⅔ cup flour | ¼ cup sugar |
| ½ cup quick-cooking oats | ¼ cup butter or margarine |

Preheat oven to 350 degrees. Butter a 9 × 9-inch baking pan or a deep 9-inch pie pan. In a large bowl, combine pudding mix, brown sugar, and flour. Add milk, water, and apples. Stir to mix. Spoon into baking pan.

For the topping, combine flour, oats, and sugar in a medium bowl. Cut in butter with a knife. Sprinkle over apple mixture in the pan. Bake for 45 to 50 minutes or until apples are tender and top is lightly browned.

*Note:* Use a cooking apple, such as Macintosh, which becomes soft when baked.

NUTRITIONAL INFORMATION PER SERVING

Calories 280; Fat 6 gm.; Protein 2 gm.; Carbohydrate 55 gm.;
Cholesterol 0 mg.; Fiber 3 gm. (high)

# *Bananas Foster*

............................... ❖ ...............................

*Bananas, brown sugar, and cinnamon—*
*a winning combination that is often prepared*
*table-side in elegant restaurants.*

❖ SERVES 4 ❖

Recipe texture: Very easy to chew

| | |
|---|---|
| ¼ cup brown sugar | ⅛ teaspoon nutmeg |
| 3 tablespoons water | 1 tablespoon butter or margarine |
| 1 tablespoon rum | 4 medium bananas |
| ¼ teaspoon cinnamon | 1 pint frozen yogurt |

In a medium saucepan, combine brown sugar, water, rum, cinnamon, and nutmeg. Bring to a boil, stirring constantly. Remove from heat and stir in butter. Peel bananas and slice diagonally. Add to sauce and toss to coat. Return to heat and cook until bubbly. Serve hot or warm with frozen yogurt.

*Note:* Some people may find bananas difficult to swallow. Cut them into very small pieces, or mash them with some sauce.

...............................

NUTRITIONAL INFORMATION PER SERVING WITH FROZEN YOGURT

Calories 230; Fat 4 gm.; Protein 3 gm.; Carbohydrate 45 gm.;
Cholesterol 15 mg.; Fiber 1.4 gm. (medium)

# Bread Pudding

❖

*A warm, comforting dessert.*

❖ SERVES 6 ❖

Recipe texture: Very easy to chew

| | |
|---|---|
| ⅓ cup raisins | ½ teaspoon cinnamon |
| 2 tablespoons brandy | ¼ teaspoon nutmeg |
| 6 thick slices day-old white bread, crusts removed | 3 eggs |
| | ⅓ cup sugar |
| 2 tablespoons butter or margarine, softened | 1 teaspoon vanilla |
| | dash salt |
| ½ cup brown sugar | 2½ cups milk |

Preheat oven to 350 degrees. Butter a 9 × 9-inch baking pan or casserole dish. Soak raisins in brandy in a custard cup. Spread bread with butter. Cut bread into cubes and lightly press into the prepared pan. Sprinkle with brown sugar, cinnamon, and nutmeg.

In a small bowl, mix eggs, sugar, vanilla, salt, milk, raisins, and brandy. Pour over bread. Place baking dish in a pan of hot water in oven. Bake for 1 hour or until knife inserted in center comes out clean. Serve warm or cool with whipped cream. Sprinkle with extra brandy if desired.

NUTRITIONAL INFORMATION PER SERVING

Calories 310; Fat 10 gm.; Protein 8 gm.; Carbohydrate 47 gm.;
Cholesterol 115 mg.; Fiber 1 gm. (medium)

# *Buttermilk Pie*

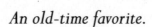

*An old-time favorite.*

Recipe texture: Easy to chew;
Soft and smooth without the crust

| | | | |
|---|---|---|---|
| 1 | cup brown sugar | 1½ cups low-fat buttermilk |
| 3 | tablespoons flour | 3 | tablespoons butter or margarine, |
| 3 | eggs | | melted |
| 1 | teaspoon vanilla | 1 | baked 9-inch pie crust |

Preheat oven to 350 degrees. In a food processor, combine all ingredients, except pie crust, and process just until blended. Pour into crust. Bake 40 to 50 minutes or until pie filling puffs and is almost set, but center still moves slightly when pan is shaken. Cool to room temperature. Refrigerate until ready to serve.

NUTRITIONAL INFORMATION PER SERVING
Calories 290; Fat 12 gm.; Protein 5 gm.; Carbohydrate 41 gm.;
Cholesterol 80 mg.; Fiber 0 gm.

# *Caramel Cheesecake*

......................................... ❖ .........................................

*This may be the smoothest, best tasting
cheesecake you have ever made.*

❖ SERVES 8 ❖

Recipe texture: Easy to chew;
Soft and smooth without the crust

**Crust**

1   cup graham cracker crumbs
¼  cup sugar

3   tablespoons butter or margarine,
    melted

**Filling**

8   ounces low-fat cream cheese,
    room temperature
4   ounces fat-free cream cheese,
    room temperature

½  cup caramel-flavored topping
3   eggs
2   tablespoons fat-free milk
2   teaspoons vanilla

**Topping**

½  cup fat-free sour cream

¼  cup caramel-flavored topping

Preheat oven to 325 degrees. In an 8-inch pie pan, combine graham
cracker crumbs with sugar and melted butter. Mix with a fork. Press
crumbs firmly in bottom of the pan and up the sides. Set aside.

*(continued)*

## *Caramel Cheesecake (continued)*

In a medium bowl, beat low-fat cream cheese, fat-free cream cheese, and caramel topping with an electric beater. Add eggs, milk, and vanilla. Beat until smooth. Pour filling into crust. Bake for 40 to 50 minutes or until light golden in color. Cool in pan for 30 minutes.

For the topping, combine sour cream and caramel topping in a small bowl. Spread on baked cheesecake. Chill in refrigerator.

NUTRITIONAL INFORMATION PER SERVING
Calories 325; Fat 15 gm.; Protein 9 gm.; Carbohydrate 39 gm.;
Cholesterol 100 mg.; Fiber 0.4 gm. (low)

# Caramel Flan

❖

*This is an easy version of the classic Spanish dessert.*

❖ SERVES 6 ❖

Recipe texture: Soft and smooth

4   eggs, slightly beaten
½  cup caramel topping, divided
dash salt
1   tablespoon rum or ½ teaspoon
    rum extract

2   cups fat-free milk
½  cup fat-free half-and-half

Preheat oven to 350 degrees. In a medium bowl, blend eggs, ⅓ cup caramel topping, salt, and rum. Gradually stir in milk and half-and-half. Place 1 teaspoon caramel topping in each of 6 custard cups. Pour custard mixture over topping. Place cups in baking pan large enough to hold the cups. Pour hot water into pan to within ½ inch of tops of cups. Bake 45 minutes or until knife inserted in the center comes out clean. Remove cups from water. Chill for 3 hours. To unmold, run knife around edge of cup, dip bottom of cup into hot water, then unmold into dessert bowl.

NUTRITIONAL INFORMATION PER SERVING
Calories 150; Fat 3 gm.; Protein 7 gm.; Carbohydrate 24 gm.;
Cholesterol 125 mg.; Fiber 0 gm.

# Cheesecake Pie

❖

*This is a cheesecake and pudding pie all in one.*

❖ SERVES 8 ❖

Recipe texture: Easy to chew;
Soft and smooth for the filling portion without the crust

1   baked 9-inch pie crust or
    meringue crust (see recipe,
    p. 195)

**Cream Cheese Filling**

8   ounces low-fat cream cheese
⅓   cup powdered sugar

¾   cup low-fat whipped topping
1   tablespoon fresh lemon juice

**Topping**

1¼ cups sugar
⅓   cup cornstarch
½   teaspoon salt
1¼ cups water

2   tablespoons butter or margarine
2   teaspoons grated lemon peel
½   cup fresh lemon juice
2   drops yellow food coloring
    (optional)

Prepare baked pie crust and set aside. In a medium bowl, combine cream cheese and sugar and beat until smooth. Fold in whipped topping and lemon juice. Spoon into pie crust and refrigerate.

In a medium saucepan, combine sugar, cornstarch, and salt. Stir in water and bring to a boil over medium heat. Cook, stirring constantly, until thickened and bubbly. Remove from heat. Stir in butter, lemon peel, and yellow coloring if desired. Gently stir in lemon juice but do not overmix. Cool to room temperature. Pour over cream cheese layer and smooth top with a knife. Refrigerate until ready to serve.

**Meringue Crust**

2   egg whites, at room temperature    1   teaspoon white vinegar
½   teaspoon vanilla    ½   cup sugar
¼   teaspoon cream of tartar
     (optional)


Preheat oven to 275 degrees. Heavily butter and lightly flour a 9-inch pie pan.

In a medium bowl, beat egg whites until firm. Add vanilla, cream of tartar, and vinegar. Continue beating and add sugar gradually. Beat until egg whites form soft peaks. Spoon into pie pan and smooth over bottom and sides of pan. Bake for 45 to 55 minutes or until lightly browned. Cool to room temperature before adding fillings.

NUTRITIONAL INFORMATION PER SERVING
Calories 350; Fat 13 gm.; Protein 4 gm.; Carbohydrate 55gm.;
Cholesterol 25 mg.; Fiber 0.7 gm. (low)

# Chess Pie

········································ ❖ ························································

*This classic dessert tastes like pecan pie without the pecans.*

❖ SERVES 8 ❖

Recipe texture: Easy to chew;
Soft and smooth for the filling portion without the crust

½  cup butter or margarine, melted
1   cup sugar
½  cup dark corn syrup
½  cup evaporated fat-free milk

3   eggs, lightly beaten
1   tablespoon flour
2   teaspoons vanilla
1   unbaked 9-inch pie crust

Preheat oven to 350 degrees. In a medium bowl, combine all ingredients except pie crust. Beat until well mixed. Pour into crust. Bake for 35 to 45 minutes or until set.

········································································································

NUTRITIONAL INFORMATION PER SERVING

Calories 400; Fat 18 gm.; Protein 4 gm.; Carbohydrate 54 gm.;
Cholesterol 100 mg.; Fiber 0.6 gm. (low)

# Chocolate Silk Pie

❖

*Melted chocolate is blended with tofu and a touch of
honey to make a smooth, delectable chocolate pie.
Don't tell anyone and they will never know there is
tofu in this dessert. If you love chocolate, this may
turn out to be your very favorite dessert.*

❖ SERVES 10 ❖

Recipe texture: Easy to chew;
Soft and smooth for the filling portion without the crust

**Crust**

1   cup graham cracker crumbs
¼   cup sugar

3   tablespoons butter or margarine

**Filling**

1   cup chocolate chips
12   ounces low-fat firm tofu
1   tablespoon honey

3   tablespoons powdered sugar
1   teaspoon vanilla
1   tablespoon brandy (optional)

In an 9-inch pie pan or a 7 × 11-inch pan, combine graham cracker
crumbs, sugar, and melted butter. Mix with a fork and press firmly in
the bottom of the pan. In a small, nonstick skillet, melt chocolate
chips over the lowest heat. Meanwhile, blend tofu, honey, sugar,
vanilla, and brandy in a food processor until very smooth. Add
melted chocolate and blend again until smooth. Pour into pan. Cover
and refrigerate.

*Note:* The pie is wonderful served with mint ice cream.

NUTRITIONAL INFORMATION PER SERVING

Calories 195; Fat 9 gm.; Protein 3 gm.; Carbohydrate 26 gm.;
Cholesterol 10 mg.; Fiber 1.6 gm. (medium)

# Classic Custard

······················ ❖ ······················

*Plain and simple.*

❖ SERVES 6 ❖

Recipe texture: Soft and smooth

butter spray
6   large eggs
½   cup sugar
¼   teaspoon salt

4   cups fat-free milk
1½ teaspoons vanilla
½   teaspoon almond extract

Preheat oven to 325 degrees. Spray a deep 2-quart casserole or soufflé dish with butter spray. In a large bowl, combine eggs, sugar, and salt. Beat well with a whisk. In a large heavy saucepan, cook milk over medium heat just until tiny bubbles form around edge, but do not boil. Remove milk from heat and gradually add to the egg mixture, stirring constantly. Stir in vanilla and almond extract. Pour into prepared dish. Place casserole in a 9 × 13-inch baking pan and add hot water to the pan to a depth of 1 inch. Bake for 50 minutes or until a knife inserted in center of custard comes out almost clean. Remove casserole from pan. Serve custard warm or chilled.

···········································································

NUTRITIONAL INFORMATION PER SERVING

Calories 180; Fat 4 gm.; Protein 11 gm.; Carbohydrate 25 gm.;
Cholesterol 180 mg.; Fiber 0 gm.

# *Cocoa Fudge Desert*

❖

*This very fudgy treat is definitely for the chocoholic.*

❖ SERVES 8 ❖

Recipe texture: Soft and smooth

| | |
|---|---|
| 1 cup flour | ¼ teaspoon salt |
| ¾ cup sugar | ½ cup fat-free milk |
| 2 tablespoons unsweetened cocoa | 2 tablespoons canola oil |
| 2 teaspoons baking powder | 1 teaspoon vanilla |

**Topping**

| | |
|---|---|
| ¼ cup unsweetened cocoa | 1¾ cups hot water |
| 1 cup brown sugar | |

Preheat oven to 350 degrees. In a large bowl, combine flour, sugar, cocoa, baking powder, and salt. Add milk, oil, and vanilla. Beat well. Spread into an ungreased 9 × 9-inch baking pan.

For the topping, combine cocoa and brown sugar in a small bowl. Sprinkle evenly over batter. Pour hot water over batter. Do not mix. Bake for 35 to 40 minutes or until cake is firm. There will be a fudge sauce at the bottom of the pan when cake is cooked. Cool in pan for 10 minutes before serving.

*Note:* This is great served with ice cream or whipped cream.

NUTRITIONAL INFORMATION PER SERVING

Calories 330; Fat 8 gm.; Protein 3 gm.; Carbohydrate 62 gm.;
Cholesterol 0 mg.; Fiber 1 gm. (medium)

# Country Apple Coffee Cake

············································ ❖ ········································

*A moist, comforting dessert.*

❖ SERVES 20 ❖

Recipe texture: Easy to chew

| | |
|---|---|
| 1  18-ounce box yellow cake mix | 1  egg, lightly beaten |
| ⅓ cup butter or margarine, softened | |

**Filling**

| | |
|---|---|
| 1  21-ounce can apple pie filling | 1  teaspoon cinnamon |
| ½ cup brown sugar | |

**Topping**

| | |
|---|---|
| 1  cup fat-free sour cream | 1  teaspoon vanilla |
| 1  egg, lightly beaten | |

Preheat oven to 350 degrees. In a large bowl, combine cake mix, butter, and egg. Stir until mixed but still crumbly. Press into a 9 × 13-inch baking pan. Pour apple pie filling over the crust. Mix brown sugar and cinnamon. Sprinkle over the top.

For the topping, combine sour cream, egg, and vanilla in a small bowl. Stir until smooth. Spoon over filling. Bake for 45 to 50 minutes or until top is set.

NUTRITIONAL INFORMATION PER SERVING

Calories 225; Fat 8 gm.; Protein 3 gm.; Carbohydrate 36 gm.;
Cholesterol 30 mg.; Fiber 0.7 gm. (low)

# Crème Caramel

❖

*A favorite comfort food from the past.*

❖ SERVES 4 ❖

Recipe texture: Soft and smooth

⅓  cup water
⅓  cup sugar
4  eggs
2  cups 2% or whole milk

⅓  cup sugar
pinch salt
1  teaspoon vanilla
1  tablespoon brandy (optional)

Preheat oven to 300 degrees. Mix water and sugar in a small heavy saucepan. Cook over medium heat until sugar dissolves and mixture turns light amber, about 8 to 10 minutes. Quickly divide hot syrup among six custard cups, tilting to coat bottoms.

In a bowl, slightly beat eggs. Add milk, sugar, salt, and vanilla without creating too many bubbles. (Bubbles on the surface do not break in the low heat needed to cook the custard.) Pour into custard cups. Place cups in a large baking pan, place the pan on an oven rack, and carefully pour hot water into the baking pan around the custard cups to a depth of about 1 inch. Bake for 55 to 60 minutes or until a knife inserted near the center comes out clean. When opening the oven door, be careful of the steam produced from the water bath. Remove cups from water. Cool and refrigerate. To serve, loosen custard from cups. Invert onto individual serving plates.

NUTRITIONAL INFORMATION PER SERVING

Calories 270; Fat 8 gm.; Protein 9 gm.; Carbohydrate 40 gm.;
Cholesterol 200 mg.; Fiber 0 gm.

# *Custard Pie*

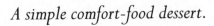

*A simple comfort-food dessert.*

❖ SERVES 8 ❖

Recipe texture: Easy to chew;
Soft and smooth for the filling portion without the crust

| | |
|---|---|
| 4 large eggs, lightly beaten | 1 teaspoon vanilla |
| 2 cups fat-free milk | ¼ teaspoon allspice |
| ½ cup fat-free half-and-half | ¼ teaspoon nutmeg |
| ½ cup sugar | 1 unbaked 9-inch pie crust |
| ¼ teaspoon salt | |

Preheat oven to 400 degrees. In a medium bowl, combine all ingredients except nutmeg and pie crust. Pour mixture into crust and sprinkle with nutmeg. Bake for 10 minutes. Turn oven to 325 degrees and bake for 45 minutes or until custard is set and knife inserted in center comes out clean.

NUTRITIONAL INFORMATION PER SERVING

Calories 205; Fat 8 gm.; Protein 6 gm.; Carbohydrate 27 gm.;
Cholesterol 90 mg.; Fiber 0.6 gm. (low)

# *Fudge Bottom Pie*

❖

*This famous recipe has been a favorite at the
University of Wisconsin campus student union for fifty years.*

❖ SERVES 8 ❖

Recipe texture: Easy to chew;
Soft and smooth for the filling portion

**Bottom**

3 ounces unsweetened chocolate
¼ cup sugar

¼ cup water
1 9-inch graham cracker pie crust

**Filling**

½ cup sugar
¼ cup cornstarch
¼ teaspoon salt

2 cups fat-free milk
3 egg yolks, lightly beaten
1 teaspoon vanilla

**Topping**

1 cup low-fat whipping cream

shaved chocolate for garnish

In a small heavy saucepan, melt chocolate over very low heat. In another small saucepan, combine sugar and water and bring to a boil. Add to melted chocolate and beat well. Spread evenly over bottom of graham cracker pie crust.

For the filling, combine sugar, cornstarch, and salt in a medium saucepan. Gradually stir in milk. Cook over medium heat, stirring constantly, until mixture boils and thickens. Cook 2 minutes more, stirring constantly. Remove from heat. Stir a small amount of hot mixture into slightly beaten egg yolks. Then slowly stir egg mixture

*(continued)*

# *Fudge Bottom Pie (continued)*

into hot milk mixture. Return to medium heat and cook another 2 minutes, stirring constantly, until mixture thickens slightly. Remove from stove, and stir in vanilla. Cool to room temperature, then pour into pie shell. Whip cream, spread over top of pie, and garnish with shaved chocolate. Refrigerate until ready to serve.

NUTRITIONAL INFORMATION PER SERVING
Calories 435; Fat 24 gm.; Protein 6 gm.; Carbohydrate 49 gm.;
Cholesterol 115 mg.; Fiber 1.6 gm. (low)

# *Key Lime Pie*

❖

*To make this authentic, use the real key limes*
*(but other limes work well also).*

❖ SERVES 8 ❖

Recipe texture: Easy to chew;
Soft and smooth for the filling portion without the crust

3   egg yolks
1   14-ounce can low-fat sweetened
    condensed milk
½   cup lime juice, fresh or bottled
2   drops green food coloring

1   8-inch baked pie crust
1   cup low-fat whipped topping
1   medium fresh lime, cut in thin
    slices

Preheat oven to 325 degrees. In large bowl, beat egg yolks with
sweetened condensed milk, lime juice, and food coloring. Pour into
prebaked pie crust. Bake 30 minutes. Cool to room temperature, then
store in the refrigerator. When ready to serve, top with whipped topping and garnish with fresh lime slices.

NUTRITIONAL INFORMATION PER SERVING

Calories 350; Fat 17 gm.; Protein 7 gm.; Carbohydrate 43 gm.;
Cholesterol 115 mg.; Fiber 0 gm.

# Lemonade Cake

❖

*This is a tart, refreshing, very moist cake.*

❖ SERVES 16 ❖

Recipe texture: Very easy to chew

1   18-ounce box lemon cake mix, with pudding in the cake
2   cups powdered sugar

1   6-ounce can frozen lemonade concentrate, thawed

Preheat oven to 350 degrees. Butter a 9 × 13-inch baking pan. Prepare and bake cake mix according to package instructions. While cake is baking, combine powdered sugar and lemonade in a small bowl. When cake is done, remove from oven and poke holes all over the cake with a meat fork. Spoon sugar and lemonade mixture over the cake and work into cake with the back of a spoon. Return to oven for 5 minutes.

*Note:* Serve with sweetened whipped cream or whipped topping.

NUTRITIONAL INFORMATION PER SERVING

Calories 205; Fat 6 gm.; Protein 1 gm.; Carbohydrate 37 gm.;
Cholesterol 20 mg.; Fiber 0 gm.

# Lemon-Lime Supreme Refrigerator Cake

❖

*A cool, refreshing, and moist dessert.*

❖ SERVES 20 ❖

Recipe texture: Soft and smooth

| | |
|---|---|
| 1 3-ounce package lime gelatin | ½ cup cold water |
| ¾ cup boiling water | 1 18-ounce box lemon cake mix |

**Topping**

| | |
|---|---|
| 1 envelope (40 grams) powdered whipped topping (yields 2 cups) | 1½ cups cold fat-free milk |
| 1 3-ounce package instant lemon pudding mix | |

Preheat oven to 350 degrees. Butter a 9 ×13-inch baking pan. In a small saucepan, dissolve gelatin in boiling water. Add the cold water and set aside at room temperature. Prepare and bake cake according to package instructions. Cool cake 20 to 25 minutes. With a meat fork, poke deep holes about 1 inch apart through top of warm cake while it is still in the pan. With a cup or pitcher, slowly pour gelatin mixture into holes. Refrigerate cake while preparing topping. Chill a deep mixing bowl and electric beaters. To prepare topping, whip topping mix, instant pudding, and cold milk until it thickens (about 5

*(continued)*

## Lemon-Lime Supreme Refrigerator Cake
### (continued)

minutes). Immediately frost cake. Store frosted cake in the refrigerator until ready to serve.

*Note:* This cake freezes well. Other flavors of gelatin such as peach or orange, can be used. Powdered whipped topping is usually found in the grocery store aisle with the gelatin desserts.

········································································································

NUTRITIONAL INFORMATION PER SERVING
Calories 180; Fat 5 gm.; Protein 2 gm.; Carbohydrate 32 gm.;
Cholesterol 1 mg.; Fiber 0 gm.

# Lemon Pudding Cake

❖

*A winning combination of soft cake and smooth pudding.*

❖ SERVES 8 ❖

Recipe texture: Easy to chew;
Soft and smooth for the pudding portion

1¼ cups sugar, divided
⅓ cup flour
⅛ teaspoon salt
1 cup fat-free milk
½ cup fresh lemon juice
2 tablespoons butter or margarine, melted

1 large egg yolk, lightly beaten
2 teaspoons grated lemon peel
4 large egg whites
¼ cup powdered sugar for garnish

Preheat oven to 350 degrees. Butter a 9-inch deep-dish pie pan. In a medium bowl, combine 1 cup sugar, flour, and salt. Make a well in the dry ingredients. Add milk, lemon juice, butter, egg yolk, and lemon peel. Whisk until smooth. In another medium bowl, beat egg whites with an electric mixer until they form soft peaks. Gradually add the remaining ¼ cup sugar, beating until glossy. Fold egg whites into batter. Spoon into pie pan. Place pie pan inside a larger shallow pan. Add enough hot water to come almost halfway up the sides of the pie pan. Bake for 30 to 40 minutes or until the top is golden. A cake layer will form on top with soft lemon pudding underneath. When ready to serve, sprinkle with powdered sugar. Serve warm.

NUTRITIONAL INFORMATION PER SERVING
Calories 210; Fat 3 gm.; Protein 3 gm.; Carbohydrate 42 gm.;
Cholesterol 35 mg.; Fiber 0 gm.

# Mandarin Orange–Pineapple Cake

❖

*This cake freezes very well. Make it ahead
and sneak it for treats, piece by piece.*

❖ SERVES 12 ❖

Recipe texture: Easy to chew

| | |
|---|---|
| 1   11-ounce can mandarin oranges in juice, undrained | 3   eggs |
| 1   18.5-ounce box yellow cake mix | ¾   cup canola oil |

**Frosting**

| | |
|---|---|
| 1   15-ounce can crushed pineapple in juice, undrained | 8   ounces low-fat whipped topping |
| 1   1.4-ounce package sugar-free instant vanilla pudding mix | |

Preheat oven to 350 degrees. Butter a 9 × 13-inch pan. In a large bowl, combine oranges, cake mix, eggs, and oil. Beat well with electric mixer. Pour into pan. Bake for 35 minutes. Cool.

For frosting, combine crushed pineapple and pudding mix in a medium bowl. Mix on low speed for 1 minute. Fold in whipped topping. Spoon on top of cake. Refrigerate until ready to serve.

NUTRITIONAL INFORMATION PER SERVING

Calories 400; Fat 20 gm.; Protein 3 gm.; Carbohydrate 53 gm.;
Cholesterol 50 mg.; Fiber 0 gm.

# Mini Cheese Cakes

❖

*An easy-to-eat, bite-size sweet treat.*

❖ SERVES 15 ❖

Recipe texture: Easy to chew;
Soft and smooth for the filling portion

15 vanilla wafer cookies
2  8-ounce packages low-fat cream
   cheese
½ cup sugar

2  eggs
¼ teaspoon nutmeg
1  teaspoon vanilla
15 fresh strawberries, optional

Preheat oven to 300 degrees. Line the cups of a muffin tin with paper liners. Place 1 cookie in each. Place all remaining ingredients except strawberries in a food processor or a medium mixing bowl. Beat until smooth. Pour mixture over cookies, filling each cup ¾ full. Bake for 35 to 40 minutes. Cool and remove from pan. Top with fresh strawberries if desired. Makes 15 mini cakes.

*Note:* Fruit from canned pie fillings, such as cherries or peaches, can be used as a topping in place of the strawberries.

NUTRITIONAL INFORMATION PER SERVING
Calories 175; Fat 7 gm.; Protein 22 gm.; Carbohydrate 5 gm.;
Cholesterol 45 mg.; Fiber 3.2 gm. (high)

# *Peach Surprise*

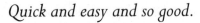

*Quick and easy and so good.*

❖ SERVES 12 ❖

Recipe texture: Easy to chew

1  21-ounce can peach pie filling
1  20-ounce can crushed pineapple,
   with juice

¾  cup butter or margarine, melted
1  18.5-ounce box yellow cake mix
butter spray

Preheat oven to 325 degrees. Butter a 9 × 13-inch baking pan. Spread pie filling in bottom of pan. Spread pineapple over peaches. In a medium bowl combine melted butter and cake mix. Blend until mixture is crumbly. Sprinkle cake mix on top of pineapple. Spray any dry spots with butter spray. Bake for 55 to 60 minutes.

*Note:* Cherry pie filling can be substituted for the peach pie filling.

NUTRITIONAL INFORMATION PER SERVING

Calories 355; Fat 16 gm.; Protein 2 gm.; Carbohydrate 51 gm.;
Cholesterol 30 mg.; Fiber 0.5 gm. (low)

# *Pistachio Pudding Pie*

❖

*Soft, smooth delight! It is also wonderful made with other pudding flavors, such as chocolate, lemon, or butterscotch.*

❖ SERVES 8 ❖

Recipe texture: Easy to chew;
Soft and smooth for the filling portion without the crust

1  8-ounce package fat-free cream cheese, at room temperature
1  tablespoon fat-free milk
1  cup powdered sugar
2  cups low-fat whipped topping, divided

1  9-inch graham cracker pie crust
2  3.4-ounce packages instant pistachio pudding mix
3  cups fat-free milk
¼  cup grated chocolate (optional)

In a small bowl, combine cream cheese, 1 tablespoon milk, and powdered sugar. Beat together. Stir in 1 cup whipped topping. Spread mixture in pie in crust. In a medium bowl, combine instant pudding mix with 3 cups milk. Beat for 2 minutes with electric mixer. Spread over cream cheese layer. Spread 1 cup whipped topping over top. Sprinkle with grated chocolate if desired.

NUTRITIONAL INFORMATION PER SERVING
Calories 395; Fat 9 gm.; Protein 8 gm.; Carbohydrate 70 gm.;
Cholesterol 10 mg.; Fiber 0 gm.

# Poached Pears with Chocolate Cranberry Sauce

❖

*An elegant and colorful dessert.*

❖ SERVES 6 ❖

Recipe texture: Easy to chew

6   cups cranberry juice cocktail
1   cup sugar
6   medium fresh pears, peeled and
    cored with stems intact

1   16-ounce can jellied cranberry
    sauce
½   cup chocolate chips

Combine cranberry juice cocktail and sugar in a large saucepan. Bring to a boil over high heat. Place pears in pan. Cover and simmer on low heat for 10 to 15 minutes or until pears are tender when pierced with a fork. Turn pears several times during cooking. Remove from heat and let cool in liquid at room temperature.

Remove pears from liquid and drain. (The cranberry juice and sugar may be refrigerated and reused. If serving it to drink, add lemon juice to taste.) Combine cranberry sauce and chocolate chips in a medium nonstick skillet. Melt over low heat, whisking occasionally, until smooth. Spoon ¼ cup of chocolate cranberry sauce into individual serving bowls. Set a pear into each bowl. Spoon remaining sauce over the pears.

NUTRITIONAL INFORMATION PER SERVING

Calories 380; Fat 4 gm.; Protein 2 gm.; Carbohydrate 84 gm.;
Cholesterol 0 mg.; Fiber 7 gm. (very high)

# *Pumpkin Bars*

❖

*Very moist and very good.*

❖ SERVES 24 ❖

Recipe texture: Very easy to chew

| | |
|---|---|
| 1  15-ounce can pumpkin | 2  teaspoons baking powder |
| 4  eggs, lightly beaten | 1  teaspoon baking soda |
| 1  cup canola oil | 2  teaspoons cinnamon |
| 2  cups sugar | 1  teaspoon pumpkin pie spice |
| 2  cups flour | |

**Frosting**

| | |
|---|---|
| 1  8-ounce package low-fat cream cheese | 4  cups powdered sugar |
| ¼  cup butter or margarine | 1  teaspoon vanilla |
| | 1  teaspoon fat-free milk |

Preheat oven to 350 degrees (325 degrees if using glass or nonstick pans). Butter two 7 × 11-inch baking pans or one 11 × 15-inch pan.

In a large bowl, combine pumpkin, eggs, oil, and sugar. Beat well. Add flour, baking powder, baking soda, cinnamon, and pumpkin pie spice. Stir until mixed. Spoon into pan. Bake 25 to 35 minutes or until a toothpick inserted in the middle comes out clean. Cool.

While bars are baking, combine frosting ingredients in a medium bowl. Beat well with electric mixer. Add extra milk if needed for desired consistency. Frost cake after it has cooled.

*Note:* Instead of 1 teaspoon pumpkin pie spice, use ½ teaspoon nutmeg, ½ teaspoon ground ginger, and ½ teaspoon ground cloves.

NUTRITIONAL INFORMATION PER SERVING

Calories 315; Fat 13 gm.; Protein 3 gm.; Carbohydrate 46 gm.;
Cholesterol 40 mg.; Fiber 0.9 gm. (low)

# Pumpkin Pie

❖

*This recipe has been a favorite in Donna's family for generations.*

❖ SERVES 8 ❖

Recipe texture: Easy to chew;
Soft and smooth for the filling portion without the crust

| | |
|---|---|
| 1   15-ounce can pumpkin | $\frac{1}{2}$   teaspoon salt |
| 1   cup sugar | $1\frac{1}{4}$ cups evaporated fat-free milk |
| $2\frac{1}{2}$ tablespoons flour | 2   eggs, well beaten |
| $1\frac{1}{2}$ teaspoons pumpkin pie spice | 1   unbaked 9-inch pie crust |
| $\frac{1}{2}$   teaspoon cinnamon | |

Preheat oven to 375 degrees. In a large bowl, mix pumpkin, sugar, flour, pie spice, cinnamon, and salt. Add milk and mix well. Add eggs and mix well. Pour into pie crust. Bake 15 minutes, then reduce oven temperature to 350 degrees. Bake another 35 to 40 minutes or until middle is set.

*Note:* Instead of 1 teaspoon pumpkin pie spice, use $\frac{1}{2}$ teaspoon nutmeg, $\frac{1}{2}$ teaspoon ground ginger, and $\frac{1}{2}$ teaspoon ground cloves.

NUTRITIONAL INFORMATION PER SERVING

Calories 270; Fat 7 gm.; Protein 6 gm.; Carbohydrate 46 gm.;
Cholesterol 50 mg.; Fiber 2.2 gm. (medium)

# *Rhubarb Bread Pudding*

❖

*If you like rhubarb, this is sure to be a favorite. It is so soft
and moist, and the flavor is absolutely wonderful.*

❖ SERVES 10 ❖

Recipe texture: Very easy to chew

| | | | |
|---|---|---|---|
| 2 | cups fat-free milk | ½ | teaspoon nutmeg |
| 2 | large eggs | ½ | teaspoon cinnamon |
| 2 | cups sugar | 5 | cups dry bread cubes |
| 2 | teaspoons vanilla | 4 | cups frozen rhubarb |

Preheat oven to 350 degrees. Grease a 7 × 11-inch baking pan. In a
large bowl, combine milk, eggs, sugar, vanilla, nutmeg, and cinnamon. Beat well. Stir in bread and rhubarb. Pour into baking pan. (Pan
will be very full.) Place pan into a 9 × 13-inch pan. Add an inch of
water in the larger pan. Bake for 60 to 70 minutes or until set in the
middle.

*Note:* It is best to use plain white bread to make the cubes. Remove
crusts, cut into cubes and dry on a baking sheet in a warm oven. It
will take about 12 slices of bread to make the 5 cups of cubes.

NUTRITIONAL INFORMATION PER SERVING

Calories 245; Fat 1 gm.; Protein 4 gm.; Carbohydrate 55 gm.;
Cholesterol 40 mg.; Fiber 1.5 gm. (medium)

# Rhubarb Crumble

❖

*If you like rhubarb, you will love this sweet, juicy dessert.*

❖ SERVES 8 ❖

Recipe texture: Easy to chew

| | |
|---|---|
| 5 cups rhubarb, sliced | ½ cup sugar |
| 1 egg, lightly beaten | |

**Topping**

| | |
|---|---|
| ¾ cup flour | 1 teaspoon cinnamon |
| 1 cup sugar | ½ cup butter or margarine |

Preheat oven to 350 degrees. Butter a 10-inch pie pan or a 9 × 9-inch baking pan. In a large bowl, combine rhubarb, egg, and sugar. Stir until mixed. Spoon into pan. In a small bowl, combine flour, sugar, and cinnamon. Add butter and cut in with a knife until mixture resembles course cornmeal. Sprinkle over rhubarb. Bake for 40 to 50 minutes or until lightly browned.

NUTRITIONAL INFORMATION PER SERVING

Calories 310; Fat 12 gm.; Protein 2 gm.; Carbohydrate 49 gm.;
Cholesterol 50 mg.; Fiber 1.5 gm. (medium)

# Rice Pudding

❖

*This is a delicious, easy way to use leftover cooked rice.*
*What a treat!*

❖ SERVES 4 ❖

Recipe texture: Very easy to chew

1   3.4-ounce package vanilla
    pudding mix
2   cups fat-free milk
2   tablespoons sugar
1   teaspoon vanilla

½   teaspoon cinnamon
⅓   cup crushed pineapple
2   cups cooked rice
⅓   cup golden raisins (optional)
½   teaspoon nutmeg for garnish

In a medium saucepan, cook pudding mix and milk according to package directions. Add sugar, vanilla, cinnamon, pineapple, and rice. Add raisins if desired. Spoon into individual bowls, cover, and refrigerate until ready to serve. Sprinkle with nutmeg.

*Note:* For a creamier consistency, use 2% or whole milk in place of fat-free milk. Add extra milk if pudding is too thick.

NUTRITIONAL INFORMATION PER SERVING
Calories 230; Fat 0 gm.; Protein 5 gm.; Carbohydrate 52 gm.;
Cholesterol 1 mg.; Fiber 0.9 gm. (low)

# *So Smooth Carrot Cake*

❖

*This easy-to-make carrot cake is extra moist and smooth
but low in calories.*

❖ SERVES 16 ❖

Recipe texture: Very easy to chew

| | |
|---|---|
| 3 large eggs | 1 6-ounce jar baby carrots |
| 1¼ cups canola oil | 1 6-ounce jar baby apricots |
| 2 cups sugar | 2 cups flour |
| 2 teaspoons cinnamon | 1 1-pound can prepared cream |
| ½ teaspoon nutmeg | cheese frosting (optional) |
| 1 teaspoon salt | |
| 2 teaspoons baking soda | |

Preheat oven to 350 degrees (325 degrees if using a glass or nonstick
pan). Grease a 9 × 13-inch baking pan. If you prefer a thinner cake,
use an 11 × 15-inch jelly roll pan. In a large mixing bowl, combine
all ingredients except flour and frosting. Beat well. Stir in flour. Pour
into baking pan. Bake 30 to 45 minutes or until a toothpick inserted
in the middle comes out clean. Cool and frost with cream cheese
frosting if desired.

NUTRITIONAL INFORMATION PER SERVING WITHOUT THE FROSTING

Calories 330; Fat 18 gm.; Protein 2 gm.; Carbohydrate 40 gm.;
Cholesterol 35 mg.; Fiber 1.1 gm. (medium)

# *Strawberry Delight*

························ ❖ ························

*This lovely and delicious dessert can also be served
as a side dish with chicken or pork.*

❖ SERVES 15 ❖

Recipe texture: Easy to chew;
Very easy to chew if strawberries are blended;
Soft and smooth, without the crust, and if strawberries are blended

¼ cup butter or margarine, melted
¼ cup brown sugar
2½ cups finely crushed pretzels
1 package sugar-free strawberry Jell-O
1½ cups boiling water
1 30-ounce package frozen sweetened strawberries, thawed

1 8-ounce package fat-free cream cheese
1 3-ounce package low-fat cream cheese
1 cup sugar
2 cups low-fat whipped topping

Preheat oven to 350 degrees. In a 9 × 13-inch glass baking pan, combine butter, brown sugar, and pretzels. Mix and pat evenly in bottom of pan. Bake for 10 minutes. Watch carefully to prevent burning. Remove from oven and cool.

In a large bowl, dissolve Jell-O in boiling water. Stir in strawberries. If desired, blend in a food processor until smooth. Chill in refrigerator until slightly thickened. Do not allow mixture to become completely set.

In a large mixing bowl, combine cream cheeses and sugar. Beat just until mixed. Fold in whipped topping. Evenly spread cream cheese mixture over pretzel crust. Spoon strawberry mixture over the cream cheese layer. Cover and chill until firm.

························

NUTRITIONAL INFORMATION PER SERVING
Calories 350; Fat 6 gm.; Protein 10 gm.; Carbohydrate 64 gm.;
Cholesterol 15 mg.; Fiber 2.3 gm. (medium)

# BEVERAGES

❖

Apple Cider Slush

Apricot-Orange Tea

Chocolate Soda

Delicious High-Calorie Malt

Mulled Cider

Orange-Vanilla Freeze

Peach Dream Drink

Peach-Strawberry Swirl

Real Fruit Slush

Sangria

Spiced Mocha Mix

Strawberry-Banana Pectin Smoothie

Strawberry-Rhubarb Freeze

Watermelon Slush

# *Apple Cider Slush*

❖

*Serve this as a slushy beverage or as a sherbet-like dessert.*

❖ SERVES 12 ❖

Recipe texture: Nectar consistency if frozen to slushy

| | |
|---|---|
| 2 cups water | 2 cups orange juice |
| 1½ cups sugar | ½ cup lemon juice |
| 4 cups apple cider or apple juice | |

In a small saucepan, combine water and sugar. Bring to a boil. Reduce heat and boil gently for 5 minutes. In a large freezer bowl, combine apple cider, orange juice, and lemon juice. Add sugar water and stir well. Cover and freeze about 2 hours or until slushy. Serve it by scraping across the top of the frozen mixture with a spoon and piling it into dessert or wine glasses.

NUTRITIONAL INFORMATION PER SERVING

Calories 155; Fat 0 gm.; Protein 0 gm.; Carbohydrate 39 gm.;
Cholesterol 0 mg.; Fiber 0 gm.

# *Apricot-Orange Tea*

❖

*This is a soothing flavor combination.*

❖ SERVES 6 ❖

Recipe texture: Thin liquid

2½ cups apricot nectar
1   cup orange juice
1   cup water
1   cinnamon stick
12  whole cloves

1   medium lemon, quartered
2   teaspoons instant tea
2   tablespoons lemon juice, or to
    taste

In a medium saucepan, combine nectar, orange juice, water, and cinnamon stick. Insert cloves into lemon quarters and add to saucepan. Bring to a boil, reduce heat, and simmer for 5 minutes. Stir in instant tea. Add lemon juice to taste.

*Note:* Continue to boil to reduce to desired liquid consistency, or use commercial thickener.

NUTRITIONAL INFORMATION PER SERVING

Calories 80; Fat 0 gm.; Protein 0 gm.; Carbohydrate 20 gm.;
Cholesterol 0 mg.; Fiber 0.7 gm. (low)

# *Chocolate Soda*

❖

*An old-fashioned favorite.*

❖ SERVES 1 ❖

Recipe texture: Nectar to honey

2  tablespoons chocolate syrup          1  cup ice cream
chilled club soda

Place chocolate syrup in tall glass. Fill glass halfway with club soda and stir. Add the ice cream, ½ cup at a time, stirring after each addition. Fill glass with club soda. Serve with a straw.

*Note:* For a thicker consistency, add extra ice cream.

NUTRITIONAL INFORMATION PER SERVING
Calories 350; Fat 13 gm.; Protein 5 gm.; Carbohydrate 53 gm.;
Cholesterol 60 mg.; Fiber 0.7 gm. (low)

# Delicious High-Calorie Malt

❖

*This is an easy way to load up on calories. If you are on a
diet, don't even lick the beaters!*

❖ SERVES 1 ❖

Recipe texture: Nectar, honey, or pudding,
depending on amount of ice cream added;
Soft and smooth

½  cup whole milk
½  cup half-and-half
2   cups ice cream, any flavor
2   tablespoons Ovaltine

1   tablespoon malted milk powder
1   package instant breakfast
    powder, any flavor

Mix all ingredients together in a food processor. Process until
smooth. Drink immediately. Save any extra in the freezer.

*Note:* This malt provides 1,000 to 1,300 calories, depending on the
ice cream you choose (ice cream ranges from 150 to 300 calories per
½-cup serving). For an extra 300 to 600 calories, add an extra cup of
ice cream.

NUTRITIONAL INFORMATION PER SERVING

Calories approx. 1100; Fat 48 gm.; Protein 26 gm.; Carbohydrate 140 gm.;
Cholesterol 180 mg.; Fiber 0 gm.

# *Mulled Cider*

························· ❖ ·························

*A traditional cold weather treat that's good any time.*

❖ SERVES 4 ❖

Recipe texture: Thin liquid, or thicken with commercial
thickener, to make the best consistency for you

| | |
|---|---|
| 4   cups apple cider | ¼  teaspoon whole cloves |
| ¼  cup brown sugar | ¼  teaspoon allspice |
| 1   cinnamon stick | ¼  teaspoon mace (optional) |

Combine all ingredients in a large pan. Heat until sugar dissolves.
Remove from heat and strain. Serve warm.

························· ❖ ·························

NUTRITIONAL INFORMATION PER SERVING

Calories 150; Fat 0 gm.; Protein 0 gm.; Carbohydrate 38 gm.;
Cholesterol 0 mg.; Fiber 1 gm. (low)

# Orange-Vanilla Freeze

❖

*Thick and smooth.*

❖ SERVES 4 ❖

Recipe texture: Soft and smooth

| | |
|---|---|
| 1 6-ounce can frozen orange juice concentrate | 1 pint vanilla ice cream |
| 2 cups fat-free milk | ¼ teaspoon cinnamon |
| | dash nutmeg |

Combine all ingredients in a food processor. Blend until smooth.

NUTRITIONAL INFORMATION PER SERVING

Calories 240; Fat 7 gm.; Protein 7 gm.; Carbohydrate 38 gm.;
Cholesterol 30 mg.; Fiber 0.4 gm. (low)

# *Peach Dream Drink*

❖ ............................................ ❖ ............................................

*This will remind you of eating peaches and cream.*

❖ SERVES 4 ❖

Recipe texture: Soft and smooth

15 ounces canned or frozen peach
slices in light syrup
1  pint vanilla ice cream

¼ cup orange juice
½ teaspoon vanilla
½ cup fat-free milk, optional

Combine all ingredients in a food processor. Blend until smooth. Add milk if needed to thin.

NUTRITIONAL INFORMATION PER SERVING

Calories 200; Fat 7 gm.; Protein 3 gm.; Carbohydrate 32 gm.;
Cholesterol 30 mg.; Fiber 1.1 gm. (medium)

# *Peach-Strawberry Swirl*

❖

*Peachy smooth and delicious.*

❖ SERVES 3 ❖

Recipe texture: Honey or nectar liquid with crushed ice;
Soft and smooth

1 peach, pitted and peeled
1 cup strawberries, fresh or frozen
1 medium banana

1 8-ounce container low-fat vanilla yogurt
5 ice cubes (optional)

Combine all ingredients in a food processor. Process until smooth.

NUTRITIONAL INFORMATION PER SERVING

Calories 115; Fat 1 gm.; Protein 5 gm.; Carbohydrate 22 gm.;
Cholesterol 5 mg.; Fiber 2 gm. (medium)

# *Real Fruit Slush*

❖

*This is good to keep on hand in the freezer.*

❖ SERVES 30 ❖

Recipe texture: Honey or nectar liquid

1   15-ounce can fruit cocktail in juice, undrained
1   15-ounce can peach slices in juice, undrained
1   8-ounce can crushed pineapple in juice, undrained
2   medium bananas, peeled and chopped

1   cup sugar
1   cup water
1   6-ounce can frozen orange juice concentrate, thawed
1   tablespoon lemon juice
lemon-lime soda, diet or regular

In a food processor or blender, combine all ingredients except lemon-lime soda. Process until smooth. If blender is small, process in several batches. Place in container with a cover and store in the freezer.

Just before serving, mash mixture with a potato masher or large spoon. For each serving, combine ¼ cup of fruit slush with soda to make it the desired consistency.

NUTRITIONAL INFORMATION PER SERVING WITHOUT THE SODA

Calories 55; Fat 0 gm.; Protein 0 gm.; Carbohydrate 14 gm.;
Cholesterol 0 mg.; Fiber 0.5 gm. (low)

# *Sangria*

......................................... ❖ .........................................

*This recipe can be increased and served
in a punch bowl for a large party.*

❖ SERVES 6 ❖

Recipe texture: Thin liquid, or thicken
to make it the best consistency for you

1   cup orange juice
1   cup lemonade
4   cups dry red wine

1   cup club soda
6   orange or lemon slices

Mix orange juice, lemonade, and red wine. Refrigerate. When ready
to serve, add club soda and garnish with orange or lemon slices.

.......................................................................................

NUTRITIONAL INFORMATION PER SERVING

Calories 140; Fat 0 gm.; Protein 0 gm.; Carbohydrate 11 gm.;
Cholesterol 0 mg.; Fiber 0; Alcohol 14 gm.

# Spiced Mocha Mix

❖

*Make your own cocoa mix.*

❖ SERVES 12 ❖

Recipe texture: Thin liquid, or thicken
to make it the best consistency for you

1   cup sugar
1   cup dry milk powder
½   cup powdered coffee creamer
½   cup cocoa powder
3   tablespoons instant coffee

½   teaspoon allspice
¼   teaspoon cinnamon
dash salt
mini marshmallows (optional)

Combine all ingredients except marshmallows and store in a covered
jar. For each serving, use 3 tablespoons of the mixture with ¾ cup
boiling water. Stir to mix and top with marshmallows if desired.

NUTRITIONAL INFORMATION PER SERVING

Calories 135; Fat 2 gm.; Protein 4 gm.; Carbohydrate 25 gm.;
Cholesterol 2 mg.; Fiber 0 gm.

# Strawberry-Banana Pectin Smoothie

························· ❖ ·························

*The fruit pectin adds fiber and smoothness.*

❖ SERVES 1 ❖

Recipe texture: Honey or nectar;
Soft and smooth

| | |
|---|---|
| 1   small banana, sliced | ⅓   cup strawberries, fresh or frozen |
| ½   cup skim milk | 2   tablespoons fruit pectin |

Place all ingredients in a blender. Process until smooth. Serve immediately.

*Note:* This drink provides 3 grams of soluble fiber. Add additional pectin for a thicker drink.

NUTRITIONAL INFORMATION PER SERVING

Calories 220; Fat 0 gm.; Protein 5 gm.; Carbohydrate 40 gm.;
Cholesterol 2 mg.; Fiber 3 gm. (high)

# *Strawberry-Rhubarb Freeze*

❖

*A winning combination!*

❖ SERVES 6 ❖

Recipe texture: Soft and smooth

| | |
|---|---|
| 2  cups sliced rhubarb | 2  cups sweetened frozen |
| ¼  cup orange juice | strawberries |
| ⅓  cup sugar | 2  teaspoons lemon juice |

In a small saucepan, combine rhubarb, orange juice, and sugar. Bring to a boil. Reduce heat and simmer for 5 to 10 minutes or until rhubarb is very tender. Place strawberries in food processor with half of the rhubarb. Process until smooth. Stir in remaining rhubarb and lemon juice. Taste mixture and add extra sugar if desired. Pour into 9 × 9-inch pan. Freeze until slushy. Scrape with spoon into serving dishes or parfait glasses.

*Note:* For a smoother consistency, add all of the rhubarb to the food processor and process until smooth.

NUTRITIONAL INFORMATION PER SERVING

Calories 70; Fat 0 gm.; Protein 0 gm.; Carbohydrate 17 gm.;
Cholesterol 0 mg.; Fiber 1.6 gm. (medium)

# *Watermelon Slush*

❖

*The perfect summer drink.*

❖ SERVES 6 ❖

Recipe texture: Honey or pudding liquid,
depending on amount of soda added;
Soft and smooth

8   cups cubed, seeded watermelon
¼   cup sifted powdered sugar
1   6-ounce can frozen lemonade
    concentrate, thawed

Mint sprigs (optional)
Club soda or 7-Up (optional)

Place watermelon in a large bowl. Cover and freeze. Combine watermelon pieces, sugar, and lemonade concentrate in a food processor. Process until smooth. Add soda for a thinner liquid. Garnish each serving with a sprig of mint.

NUTRITIONAL INFORMATION PER SERVING

Calories 100; Fat 0 gm.; Protein 1 gm.; Carbohydrate 24 gm.;
Cholesterol 0 mg.; Fiber 0.7 gm. (low)

# Dietary Supplements

ere are some examples of currently available dietary supplements to boost your intake of protein, calories, and fiber.

| Product | Serving Size | Calories | Protein (gm) | Fat (gm) | Carbohy-drate (gm) | Special Characteristics |
|---|---|---|---|---|---|---|
| Boost (Mead Johnson) | 8 oz | 240 | 10 | 4 | 4 | High calories and protein, low fat |
| Boost Hi Pro (Mead Johnson) | 8 oz | 240 | 14.5 | 6 | 33 | Higher protein |
| Boost Plus (Mead Johnson) | 8 oz | 360 | 14 | 13 | 45 | High calories and protein |
| Boost High Fiber (Mead Johnson) | 8 oz | 240 | 10 | 4 | 42 | 3 grams fiber |
| Boost Breeze | 8 oz | 160 | 8 | 0 | 31 | Juice based with milk protein; lactose-free |
| Carnation Instant Breakfast | 1 packet | 130 | 5 | 0 | 28 | Mix with milk of your choice |
| Choice-dm (Mead Johnson) | 8 oz | 220 | 10.6 | 10 | 24 | Balanced for diabetics with lower carbohydrate |

| Product | Serving Size | Calories | Protein (gm) | Fat (gm) | Carbohy-drate (gm) | Special Characteristics |
|---|---|---|---|---|---|---|
| Enlive (Ross) | 8 oz | 300 | 10 | 0 | 65 | Clear liquid (not creamy) with fruit flavors; high carbohydrate |
| Ensure (Ross) | 8 oz | 250 | 9 | 6 | 40 | Lactose- and milk-free; high protein |
| Ensure Plus (Ross) | 8 oz | 360 | 13 | 11 | 50 | Lactose- and milk-free; high calorie and protein |
| Ensure High Protein (Ross) | 8 oz | 230 | 12 | 6 | 31 | Lactose- and milk-free; high protein |
| Ensure Light (Ross) | 8 oz | 200 | 10 | 3 | 33 | Lower in calories; low fat |
| Ensure with Fiber (Ross) | 8 oz | 260 | 9.4 | 8.8 | 38 | Lactose- and milk-free; high fiber (3.4 gm) |
| Equate (Wal-Mart) | 8 oz | 250 | 9 | 9 | 33 | Low cost |
| Equate Plus (Wal-Mart) | 8 oz | 360 | 13 | 13 | 47 | High calorie, low cost |
| Glucerna (Ross) | 8 oz | 240 | 10 | 13 | 20 | Balanced for diabetics |
| Lipisorb (Mead Johnson) | 8 oz | 240 | 8.4 | 11.5 | 25 | 85 percent of fat is from medium-chained-triglyceride (MCT) oil; marketed for persons with fat malabsorption. |

| Product | Serving Size | Calories | Protein (gm) | Fat (gm) | Carbohy-drate (gm) | Special Characteristics |
|---------|--------------|----------|--------------|----------|---------------------|-------------------------|
| Magnacal (Sherwood) | 8 oz | 500 | 17.5 | 20 | 62 | Very high-calorie; vanilla flavor only |
| Osmolite HN | 8 oz | 250 | 9 | 9 | 34 | High protein; bland, plain flavor |
| Pulmocare (Ross) | 8 oz | 355 | 14.8 | 21 | 25 | For pulmonary patients |
| Resource (Novartis) | 8 oz | 250 | 9 | 6 | 40 | Lactose- and milk-free |
| Resource Plus (Novartis) | 8 oz | 360 | 13 | 11 | 52 | Lactose- and milk-free; high calories and protein |
| Resource Diabetic (Novartis) | 8 oz | 250 | 15 | 11 | 23 | Lower carbohydrates |
| Resource Fruit Beverage (Novartis) | 8 oz | 180 | 9 | 0 | 36 | Clear liquid |
| Resource Thickened Juice— Honey or Nectar Consistency* (Novartis) | 8 oz | 160–180 | 0–1 | 0 | 39–47 | Lactose- and milk-free; thickened liquid (not creamy) with fruit flavors |
| Resource Dairy Thick—Honey or Nectar Consistency (Novartis) | 8 oz | 180–190 | 8 | 5 | 26–28 | Creamy; made with 2% thickened milk; has 50 percent more calcium than milk |
| Resource Thickened Coffee* (Novartis) | 8 oz | 36–40 | 0 | 0 | 9–10 | |
| Resource Thickened Tea (Novartis) | 1 packet (14 gm) | 50 | 0 | 0 | 13 | Add water, stir, and serve |

| Product | Serving Size | Calories | Protein (gm) | Fat (gm) | Carbohydrate (gm) | Special Characteristics |
|---|---|---|---|---|---|---|
| Resource Thickened Cocoa (Novartis) | 1 packet (34 gm) | 130 | 1 | 1.5 | 30 | Add water, stir, and serve |
| Resource Thickened Water Honey or Nectar Consistency* (Novartis) | 8 oz | 35–40 | 0 | 0 | 9–10 | Thickened water with a slight lemon flavor |
| Resource Just for Kids (Novartis) | 8 oz | 237 | 7 | 12 | 26 | Also available with fiber |
| ScandiShakes (Scandipharm) | 3 oz powder (with 1 cup whole milk) | 600 | 12 | 30 | 70 | Very high calorie; high protein and fat; lactose-free available |
| Slim Fast Ultra | 11 oz | 220 | 10 | 3 | 40 | Similar to Ensure Light, plus 5 gm fiber |
| Slim Fast with Soy Protein | 11 oz | 220 | 7 | 1 | 44 | Soy protein with 5 gm fiber |
| Sport Shake (Mid-America Dairymen) | 11 oz | 430 | 13 | 13 | 63 | High-calorie and high-protein |
| Walgreen's Nutritional Drink | 8 oz | 250 | 9 | 6 | 40 | Lower cost |
| Walgreen's Nutritional Supplement Plus | 8 oz | 360 | 13 | 13 | 47 | Lower cost |

*Another brand of thickened juice, water, and coffee is NutraBalance, available from Sysco Corporation.

*Note:* Check labels for new formulations and look for new products on the market. These products and other generic store-brand products may be purchased in pharmacies, drug stores, grocery stores, and discount stores.

Some of the products mentioned can be ordered directly from the companies and shipped to your home. Phone numbers as of this writing are:

| | | |
|---|---|---|
| Mead Johnson | (800) | 247-7893 |
| Nestle Foods | (800) | 289-7313 |
| Novartis Nutrition | (800) | 828-9194 |
| Ross Labs | (800) | 544-7495 |
| ScandiPharm | (800) | 4-SCANDI (472-2634) |

The following are some additional commercial products available to add extra calories, fat, protein, or fiber to your diet. They are in powder or liquid form, and can be incorporated into food or drinks.

- Polycose or Sumacal (a flavor-neutral carbohydrate), 23 calories per tablespoon
- Nestle's Additions (a flavor-neutral food enhancer) 100 calories and 6 grams of protein per scoop (19 grams)
- Lipomul, 6 calories per cc, or 90 calories per tablespoon
- MCT Oil (Medium-chained-triglyceride oil), 8 calories per cc or 116 calories per tablespoon
- Resource Protein Powder, 6 grams protein per scoop (7 grams)
- Resource Benefiber, 16 calories, 4 grams carbohydrate, 3 grams fiber per tablespoon

# APPENDIX B

# Resources and Product Information

## Eating and Drinking Adaptive Devices and Utensils

**AliMed Inc.**
297 High Street
Dedham, MA 02026
(800) 225-2610
Fax: (800) 437-2966
E-mail: info@alimed.com
Internet: www.alimed.com

AliMed sells dysphagia-related products ranging from diet modification recipes and dysphagia assessment tools to feeding and swallowing aids.

**Elder eStore**
4057 Highway 9 North, Dept. 128
Howell, NJ 07731
Fax (732) 363-8920
E-mail: cs@elderestore.com
Internet: www.elderestore.com

Elder eStore has a wide range of adaptive utensils and kitchen equipment that can make eating easier.

**Enrichments Sammon-Preston, Inc. Catalog**
P.O. Box 5071
Bolingbrook, IL 60440
(800) 323-5547

Enrichments catalog specializes in adaptive kitchen utensils and devices.

**Providence Spillproof**
P.O. Box 40672
Providence, RI 02940
(888) 843-5287
Fax: (401) 521-0522
E-mail: info@kcup.com
Internet: www.kcup.com

Providence Spillproof specializes in different adaptive cups, including Nosey Cups and the Kennedy spillproof drinking cup.

**WisdomKing.com Inc.**
2066 Mar Azul Way
Carlsbad, CA 92009
(877) 931-9693

Fax: (760) 727-6479
E-mail (customer service):
customerservice@wisdomking.com
E-mail (billing):
billing@wisdomking.com
www.wisdomking.com/line250.html

WisdomKing.com sells a wide range of products for people with dysphagia and for clinicians treating people with dysphagia. These products include rubber spoons, Clip-On food guards, dysphagia cups, books for clinicians, and Thick & Easy food thickener.

## Educational Materials

**Dysphagiaonline.com**
Internet:
www.dysphagiaonline.com

Dysphagiaonline.com provides patients and professionals who have an interest in dysphagia with "one-stop-shop" access to patient, professional, and product information.

**Dysphagia Resource Center**
Internet: www.dysphagia.com

This site provides links to an abundance of other web sites that contain information regarding swallowing and swallowing disorders including vendor lists, organizations and foundations, Internet journals, reference lists, book lists, and book reviews.

**MEDLINEplus: Dysphagia**
National Institute on Deafness and Other Communication Disorders

National Institutes of Health
31 Center Drive, MSC 2320
Bethesda, MD 20892
Internet: www.nlm.nih.gov/
medlineplus/dysphagia.html

This site provides a wealth of dysphagia information from the National Institute on Deafness and Other Communication Disorders, including health information, research funding, news, and publications.

## Food Products and Thickeners

**4webmed**
2805 North Commerce Parkway
Miramar, FL 33025
Toll-free: (877) 493-2633
E-mail:
swallowinfo@4webmed.com
Internet: www.4webmed.com

4webmed specializes in locating and ordering specialized nutritional products, making it easy for patients to place one order for all their nutritional supplement requirements. They carry both frozen and shelf-stable products, including products from the following manufacturers: American Nutriceuticals, Diamond Crystal, Novartis, Hormel, Cliffdale Farms, and Ross Nutra/Balance.

**Martin Brothers Nutrition Services**
406 Viking Road
Cedar Falls, IA 50613

(800) 847-2404
E-mail: jshephard@martinsnet.com
Internet:    www.martinsnet.com/
nutprodguides.asp

Martin Brothers Nutrition Services sells many dysphagia food products, including thickened supplements and beverages, thickeners, puréed foods, high-calorie/high-protein supplements, high-fiber supplements, a lactose-free supplement, and protein and calorie additives. They also are known for their wide selection of finger foods.

**Hormel Health Labs**
E-mail: hhl@hormel.com
Internet:
www.hormelhealthlabs.com

Hormel Health Labs provides an extensive group of products for individuals with swallowing disorders including Cliffdale Farms texture-modified foods, Thick & Easy thickener, puréed meats, and instantized pasta.

**Novartis Medical Nutrition**
(800) 333-3785
Internet:
www.novartisnutrition.com

- Resource ThickenUp is an instant food thickener supplemented with vitamins and minerals. It dissolves rapidly in cold and hot substances and does not thicken over time.
- Resource Protein Instant is a concentrated, unflavored protein powder that can be added to beverages and soft foods.
- Resource Hydration Gelatin is a snack that provides fluids in a gelatin form. It provides 120 calories, 4 grams of protein, and 100 cc of fluid per ½-cup serving. It has a smooth, puddinglike consistency and comes in several flavors.
- Resource Solutions Puréed Egg & Toast Mix is a shelf-stable mix that combines the nutrition of puréed eggs and toast in a single serving. Mixed with hot water, it provides 200 calories and 10 grams of protein in a ½-cup serving. It has a cohesive texture, better than standard scrambled eggs, which can fall apart in the mouth and are difficult to control and swallow.
- Resource Puréed Bread Mix is a shelf-stable mix that offers a safe way to enjoy bread on a soft-and-smooth diet. It has a good bread flavor and can be molded for a "real bread" look. It has a smooth, cohesive consistency and provides 80 calories, 3 grams of protein, and 3 grams of fiber per serving.

**DC Distributors Inc.**
P.O. Box 224
Amherst, NY 14226
(716) 877-6534
Toll-free: (800) 827-6763
E-mail: dc@dcdistributors.com
Internet: www.dcdistributors.com

DC Distributors Inc. sells Thicken Right food thickeners as well as products that add vitamins and nutrition to food and products that help shape and add texture to food. In addition, they provide tips for preparing beverages, fruits, vegetables, and meats.

## Kitchen Equipment and Supplies

### Chef's Catalog
P.O. Box 620048
Dallas, TX 75262
Toll-Free: (800) 884-2433
Fax: (972) 401-6400
Internet: www.chefscatalog.com

Chef's Catalog sells an array of cookware, kitchen tools, and kitchen electrical equipment. They have a particularly good selection of blenders, juicers, and food processors.

## Professional Organizations

### American Academy of Otolaryngology-Head and Neck Society (AAO-HNS)
One Prince Street
Alexandria, VA 22314
(703) 836-4444
TTY: (703) 519-1585
Fax: (703) 683-5100
E-mail: entinfo@aol.com
Internet: www.entnet.org

### American Dietetic Association
Internet: www.eatright.org

### American Occupational Therapy Association, Inc.
4720 Montgomery Lane
P.O. Box 31220
Bethesda, MD 20824
(301) 652-2682
Fax: (301) 652-7711
Internet: www.aota.org

### American Speech-Language-Hearing Association
10801 Rockville Pike
Rockville, MD 20852
Voice/TTY: (301) 897-5700
Toll free: (800) 638-8255
E-mail (general):
actioncenter@asha.org
E-mail (for topics related to speech-language pathology including dysphagia):
slpinfo@asha.org
Internet: www.asha.org

This site describes problems in the oral, pharyngeal, and esophageal phases of swallowing; causes; general signs; results; and the role of the speech-language pathologist.

### National Cancer Institute (NCI)
Building 31, Room 10A16
National Institutes of Health
Bethesda, MD 20892
Toll-free: (800) 422-6237
Voice/TTY: (800) 332-8615
Internet: www.nci.nih.gov

### National Institute of Diabetes and Digestive and Kidney Diseases (NIDDK)
Building 31, Room 9A04
National Institutes of Health

Bethesda, MD 20892
(301) 496-3583
Internet: www.niddk.nih.gov

## Support Organizations

**American Stroke Association**
Internet:
www.strokeassociation.org

**Amyotrophic Lateral Society Association**
27001 Agoura Rd.
Suite 150
Calabasas Hills, CA 91301
Toll-free: (800) 782-4747
Fax: (818) 880-9006
Internet: www.alsa.org

**National Multiple Sclerosis Society**
1-800-Fight-MS (1-800-344-4867)
The National Multiple Sclerosis Society
733 Third Avenue
New York, NY 10017
Internet: www.nationalmssociety. org

**National Parkinson Foundation, Inc.**
Bob Hope Parkinson Research Center
Bob Hope Road
Miami, FL 33136
(305) 243-6666
Toll-free national: 1-800-327-4545
Fax: (305) 243-4403
E-mail: mailbox@parkinson.org
Internet: www.parkinson.org

**Support for People with Oral and Head and Neck Cancer (SPOHNC)**
Yul Brynner Head and Neck Cancer Foundation
P.O. Box 250582
Charleston, SC 29425
(843) 792-6624
Fax: (843) 792-0546
Internet: www.spohnc.org

# Index